First Steps

A Guide to Motor Skills in the First Year

Amanda Husain, PT, DPT, PCS

Disclaimer: This Book is for Educational and Informational Purposes Only.

This book is dedicated to my husband for his support and encouragement and to my son for his inspiration.

Thank you to all my mentors and "editors" along the way!

About the Author

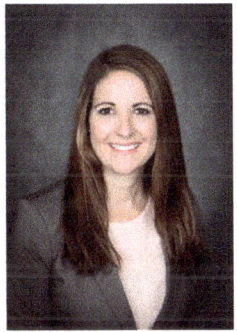

Dr. Amanda Husain, PT, DPT, PCS, is a board-certified pediatric physical therapist with over a decade of experience in both inpatient and outpatient pediatric hospital settings. She earned her B.S. in Exercise Physiology from Ohio University in 2011 and her Doctor of Physical Therapy degree from Washington University in St. Louis in 2014. Throughout her career, she has worked with children and families at leading institutions including Boston Children's Hospital, Children's Hospital of Orange County, and MemorialCare Miller Children's & Women's Hospital Long Beach.

Passionate about helping children move, play, and grow, Dr. Husain believes that healthy movement habits start early. Inspired by her experiences as a mother, NICU parent, and lifelong athlete—having competed as a collegiate swimmer and Olympic trials qualifier—she strives to make information about movement and health accessible to parents, children, teens, and young adults alike.

For more information including future content, additional tips, and recommendations on toys please visit peakplaying.org.

Gross Motor Skill Checklist

Most infants should reach the listed motor skills by the age above.

6 Months

Rolling back to tummy
Rolling tummy to back

9 Months

Sitting without support

10 Months

Crawling

12 Months

Standing
Cruising

15 Months

Walking

Table of Contents

Introduction

"The journey of a thousand miles begins with a single step."

LAO TZU

Watching your baby take their first steps is one of the many highlights we experience as a parent. It's the culmination of countless hours of practice by your little one that brings about a new level of freedom and exploration. In this book, my hope is to provide parents and caregivers with ideas to help foster development in strength, coordination, and motor skill acquisition through play.

Throughout my career as a pediatric physical therapist, I have noticed a common theme surrounding the importance of prevention. It isn't just rehabilitating an infant after their open-heart surgery; it's encouraging safe tummy time, so they don't lose their strength and develop flatness of their head. It isn't simply providing safe exercises for a child undergoing chemotherapy and radiation for their cancer, it's preventing the deconditioning from their brutal treatment regimen. It isn't only getting motion back in a joint for a child with rheumatoid arthritis, it's teaching them joint protection strategies to prevent further damage. It isn't merely getting the child who has been unconscious in the intensive care unit walking again, it's preventing bedsores, pneumonias, and deconditioning. It isn't purely rehabilitating the star soccer player who tore their ACL, it's instructing them in proper ways to cut and pivot to avoid reinjury. Time and again, the focus is on prevention, and this is especially true for my infant clients.

Physical therapists are privy to crucial information on handling to optimize infant motor skills. This knowledge can prevent a wide range of impairments and more parents should have access. Throughout my career I have treated infants with conditions that could have been easily avoided if their caregivers had these simple tips sooner.

A 2-year-old child presents to me with persistent toe walking. I take a history of their development and daily activities and learn they spent a lot of time in a "walker" hoping to strengthen their legs, but primarily using their toes to propel themselves around. A 6-month-old infant has a flat head that is going to require a helmet for remolding. Turns out they also have reflux and hate tummy time, so most of their day they are on their back reclined in a swing or bouncer. A 10-month-old presents with parent concerns regarding an asymmetrical crawl without any other delays or asymmetries. The mother is concerned it is a sign of something bigger and has been stressed about it for weeks. A 15-month-old arrives with concerns of delayed motor skills. The toddler isn't walking yet. The grandmother tells me he stopped trying to walk after falling while walking to her after she backed up, trying to get him to walk further. Now he is fearful to try again. These stories are just a small sample of the clients who have come to me over the years with concerns that could have been prevented if only they had access to the information in this book.

The inspiration to enlighten other parents came after my own son was born. I went into preterm labor at 33 weeks of pregnancy, later found to be caused by a placental abruption. This means that my placenta became separated from the uterus and the blood supply became interrupted. A placental abruption can cause the mother to lose too much blood, leading to the infant receiving an inadequate blood supply. The possible result is significant injury and death to both the mother and baby.

My son was born at 34 weeks--6 weeks early. He spent 2 weeks in the neonatal intensive care unit, then was able to come home with us. I found that having the privilege of my physical therapist knowledge, I was able to prevent many issues that may have arisen due to my son's birth risk factors. I want more parents to have that privilege.

Before you move forward, I want to provide a disclaimer that there is no link between early walking and kids getting a college sports scholarship, going pro, or winning an Olympic gold medal. There are so many factors that can affect a child's motor skill development. From body and head size to personality differences, each child is unique and should not be expected to do the exact same things as their peers. Avoid the temptation to compare your child to their siblings, your friend's children, and other babies at the playground. Take comfort in providing safe opportunities to explore for your child, and perhaps incorporating some of the activities in this book.

When you do have concerns, please speak with your child's pediatrician. In some cases, a referral to a pediatric physical therapist is warranted. Additionally, please note this book is written for parents of children who do not have a known disability or other diagnosis that requires close physical therapist direction.

Chapter 1

Floor Time

One of the most important ways to get your baby moving
and exploring is floor time. Being on the floor allows
freedom of movement and allows your baby to interact
with their world. Floor time can begin immediately and
helps babies to stretch and strengthen their muscles,
develop motor control and coordination, and learn about
their world.

After being curled in the womb for the past 9 months with increasingly less space, newborns come out with tight flexor muscles. These are the muscles that bring the arms and legs inward toward the tummy. Allowing them time on the floor facilitates stretching through gravity. Additionally, infants kick their legs and bat their arms a lot when they are free to move, which helps strengthen the extensor muscles and stretch out the tight flexor muscles. They start to learn that if they move their arm or leg in a certain way they may hit a toy, making a fun sound, and if they turn their head, they can see their loving parents.

For the first few months, infants can only see 8-15 inches away. They love faces and high contrast toys such as those with black, white, and red images. Babies turn their head to your voice and to a rattle. You can use these strategies to get your baby to start turning their head, visually scanning their environment (looking up, down, and side to side), and lifting their head while on their tummy. Preferred sounds and visual input encourage kicking and batting of the arms. There are even little rattles you can attach to the wrists and ankles! Eventually, as your baby gets stronger and more coordinated, they will start to try moving and reaching toward these preferred toys.

To safely support floor time, it is important to identify a clear space for your baby that is free of potential hazards. A play yard or fence and mat can be very helpful. There are also numerous baby gyms you can find at stores and online. You can start floor time on day one of life.

Look for times when your baby can tolerate being unswaddled while awake, calm, and alert. While playing, look for signs of stress such as hiccupping, yawning, sneezing, disorganized activity, crying, and falling asleep. If your baby is showing these behaviors, decrease stimulation until they achieve a calm, alert state. Strategies to help decrease stimulation can include lowering the lights, patting, gentle pressure of your hand on the tummy, or decreasing sound. To resume a quiet state if these strategies aren't working, stop floor time and try swaddling, holding, shushing, and rocking. Start with 5-10 minute bouts of floor time and watch your baby's cues as mentioned previously. Most infants will not tolerate more than 20-30 minutes of physical activity at a time for the first few months.

I have given this advice to parents throughout my career, and it was easy to accomplish in a therapy facility set up for babies. However, when it was time to start floor time with my own son, I will admit I was nervous! He was so very small, and he enjoyed being swaddled and held. I was afraid he would be uncomfortable and overstimulated, especially since he was born prematurely.

We started floor time when he was adjusted to a newborn age, after what should have been his birthday. We started small, just 5-10 minutes at a time on a large mat set up in a room closed off from our pet cat and clear of clutter. He had a play gym with hanging toys, high contrast books, and mirror toys. We used rattles and our smiling faces to entice him to look around and get him kicking and batting his arms. It was amazing! He was too little to show us his cute smile, but he was calm and focused. After those first couple of days, it became easier to get him his play time on the floor.

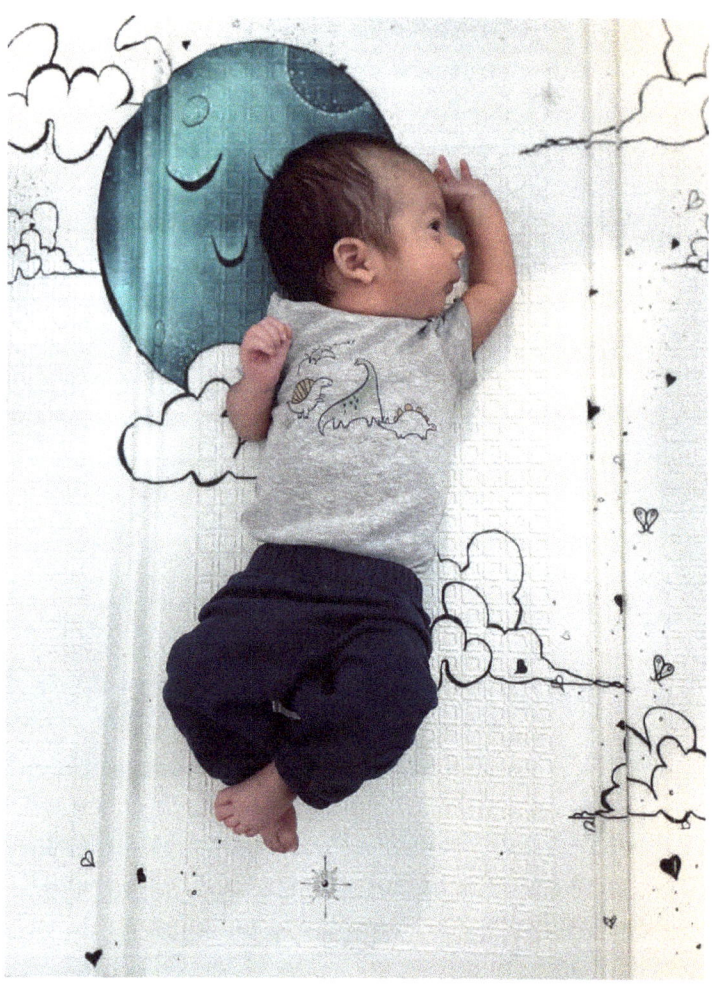

Newborns are born with their arms and legs flexed. Being on the floor allows them to move freely into extension and stretch their muscles.

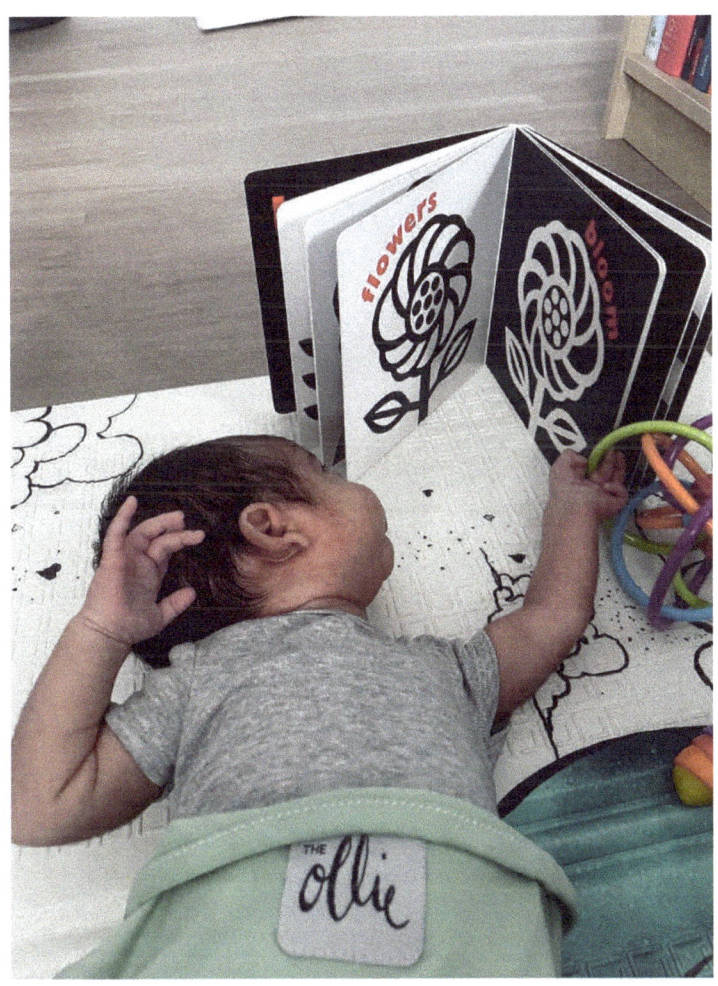

Putting black, white, and red contrast books in different locations, and giving easy rattles to hold will help encourage your baby to explore with vision and hearing, encouraging independent movement.

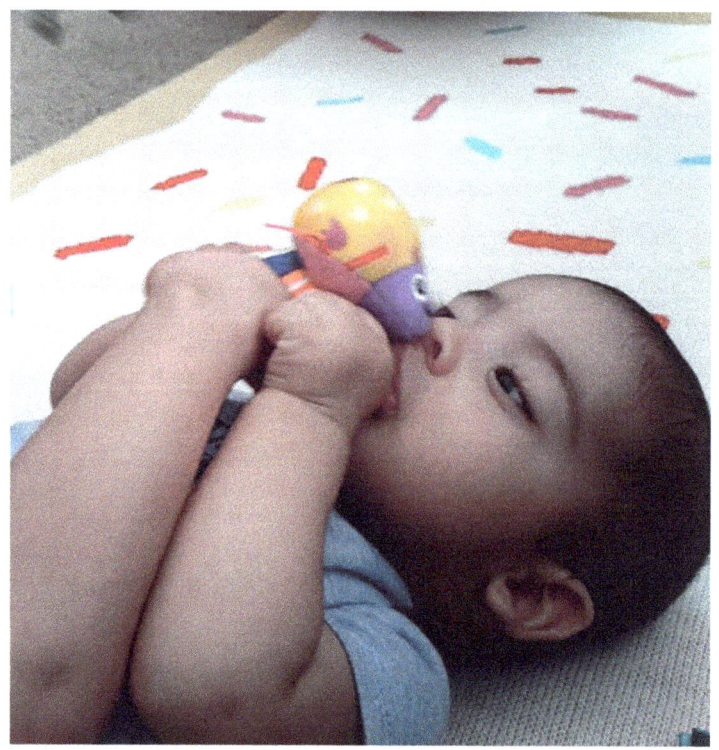

Rattles on the feet entice babies to reach to their toes, strengthening their abdominal muscles. The sounds encourage increased kicking at younger ages as well!

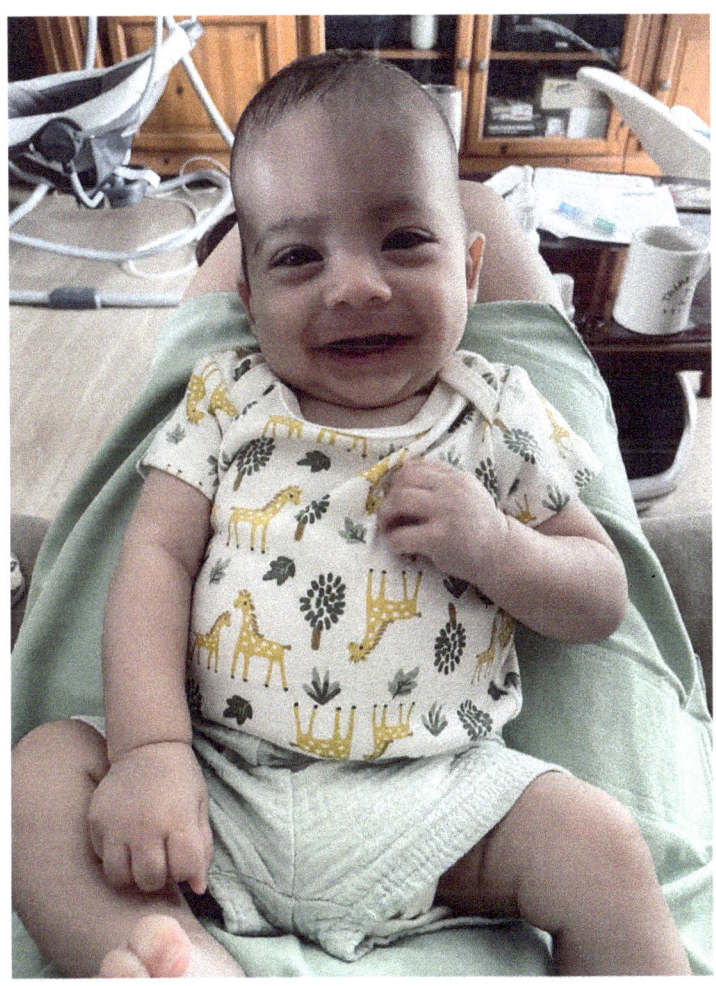

Positioning your baby on your legs encourages social engagement while allowing free movement.

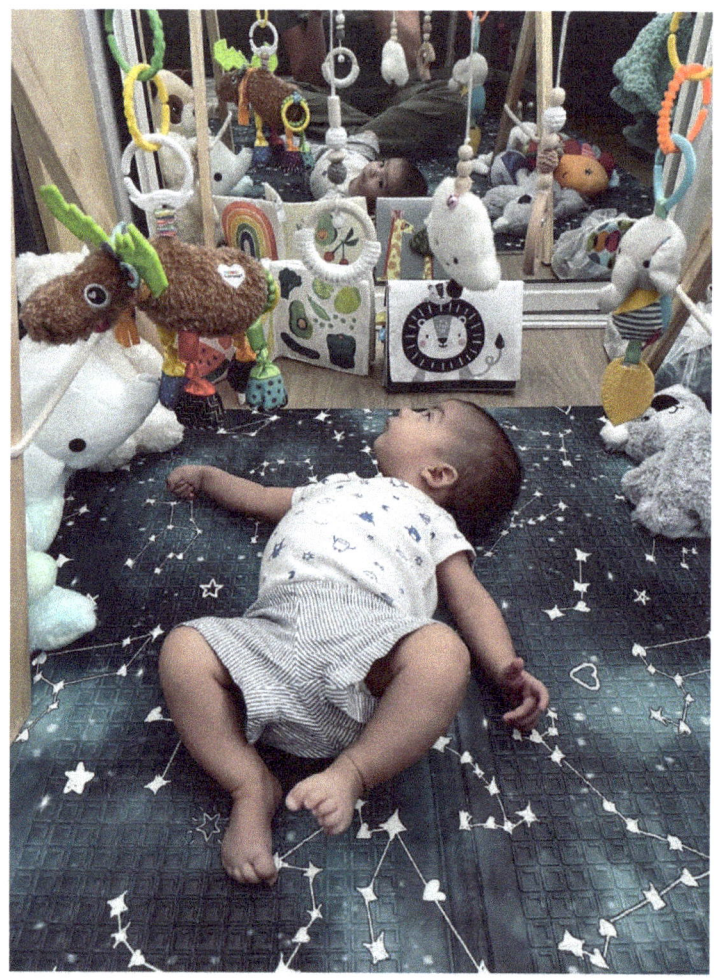

Position toys in different locations to encourage visual scanning. Alternate which direction your baby looks to promote symmetrical skill acquisition and even head shape. Your baby might initiate turning their body, preparing to roll.

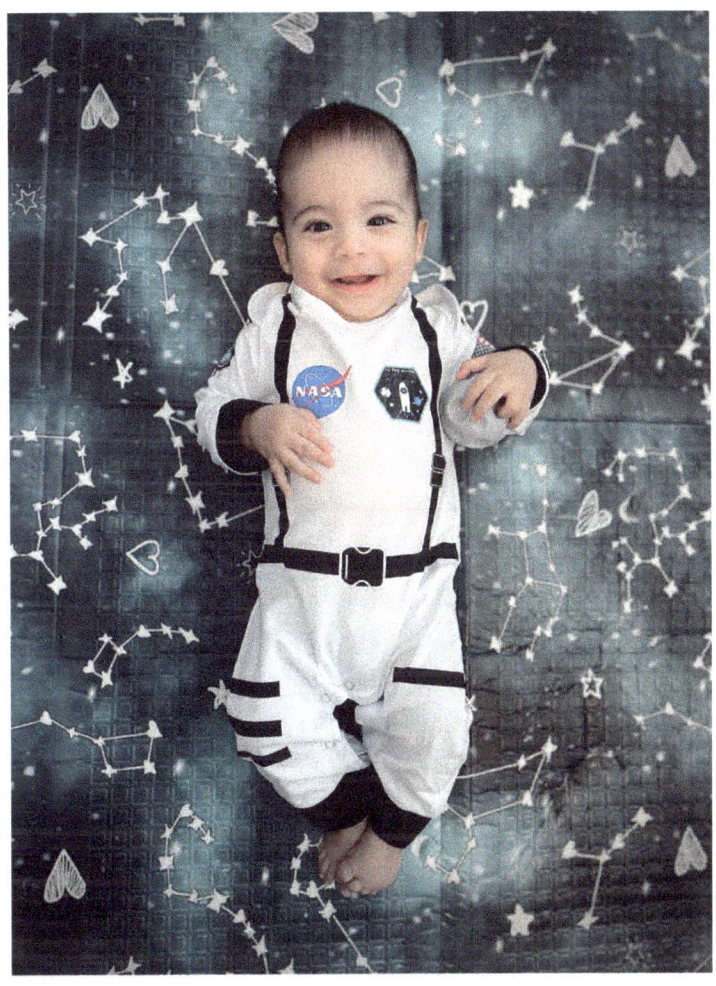

Floor time is fun!

Chapter 2

Tummy Time

Ask any pediatric physical therapist what the most important activity is for babies, and they'll probably answer tummy time. It is an important skill because it helps stretch out the flexor muscles, strengthen the extensor, core, and arm muscles, develop head control, develop hand-eye coordination, maintain a round head and prevent flat spots from developing, and it can even help with gas relief. Tummy time can start immediately along with floor time.

After the crucial "Back to Sleep" initiative to reduce sudden infant death, infants started spending less time on their tummies. Tummy time is safe when your baby is awake, calm, and alert but should be avoided during sleep and nap time to reduce the risk of death. If it is done regularly when your baby is awake, you can prevent conditions like torticollis (a tightness of specific neck muscles causing babies to tilt and rotate their head) and plagiocephaly (flat spot on the head). It is worth noting that torticollis and plagiocephaly can be caused while baby is in the womb. If this is the case, tummy time may not help prevent it but it can help treat the conditions especially if accompanied with physical therapy.

Additional barriers to floor and tummy time include difficulty finding safe space and uninterrupted time. "Container" devices have become widely available to provide safe and easy spaces for caregivers to place their infants while attending to other children, work, and other necessary tasks. "Container" devices include swings, bouncers, and infant carriers. These can be necessary for parents but can limit the amount of time an infant gets to freely move and explore. In general, parents should limit time in these devices to 15-minute bouts. Infant carriers can be a reasonable alternative to prevent plagiocephaly but will not allow free movement for the arms and legs.

Tummy time can also be challenging for some infants. Reflux is a common condition that can make being on the tummy uncomfortable. Sometimes the position can induce spit ups, especially when done after a feeding. Infants with a larger head size also may struggle with the position since it takes more effort to lift and clear their head. Lastly, babies can find it less enjoyable if they can't easily engage with their toys or preferred activities in tummy time. Being prepared with strategies for alternative positioning and engagement is the key to success.

Keep tummy time consistent and fun. The goal is to build up to at least an hour of tummy time per day, but you can break it up into small 5-minute increments or to your baby's tolerance. It is important to try and make the position comfortable and fun. This ensures good motor learning can happen in the brain and will help you be successful in increasing your baby's endurance to the position.

Some alternative positions include over a "u" shaped pillow or towel roll, on parent's chest (the more you recline, the more challenging it will be for your baby), and carried in the arms (think "airplane"). The airplane position cannot be done until your baby has some head control. The goal is to get your baby to lift their head up and look around. In the "airplane" position, your baby will not get the benefit of putting weight through their arms or stretching out the front of their legs. You can work on these with skills such as prop sitting, kneeling with arms extended on a support, and side sitting with arm down to the side. These alternative arm weight bearing positions are not appropriate until your baby has head control.

Toys and funny faces that are easily viewed while on the tummy will keep the activity meaningful and engaging to your baby. A nice soft mirror toy you can lay flat or prop up is a wonderful option. High contrast books and soft crinkle toys can be easy options for young infants. Smiling faces of parents and siblings, and pets, are some of the most motivating options. Bonus points for singing and funny noises!

Our son ended up loving tummy time, but initially the position was uncomfortable for him. He had reflux, which contributed to his discomfort. We tried spacing tummy time out from when he would feed, but it didn't seem to make enough of a difference for him and it made it difficult to get tummy time in since he ate so often! He arched his back a lot due to his reflux and coupled with him not liking the position, he learned quickly to roll onto his back.

Since we couldn't get a lot of good tummy time initially, we made sure to spend a lot of time with him on our chests. We would gradually recline ourselves on the couch to get him to lift his head against gravity. The first time he lifted his head and turned to try and look at us will stay with me forever! It was so rewarding. We did not use a towel roll or "u" shaped pillow often, but they can be very useful. They help shift the body weight back onto the pelvis to allow babies to lift their head easier. You can also use your hand to accomplish this, which is often what I did.

Our son ended up on medication to help manage his reflux and after that, tummy time was easier for him. Perhaps he had more strength in his neck by then, but he became a tummy time champion! He would check himself out in the mirror, try to reach for his crinkle book, and once he hit 3 months old, he gave us the most winning gummy smiles for our goofy noises.

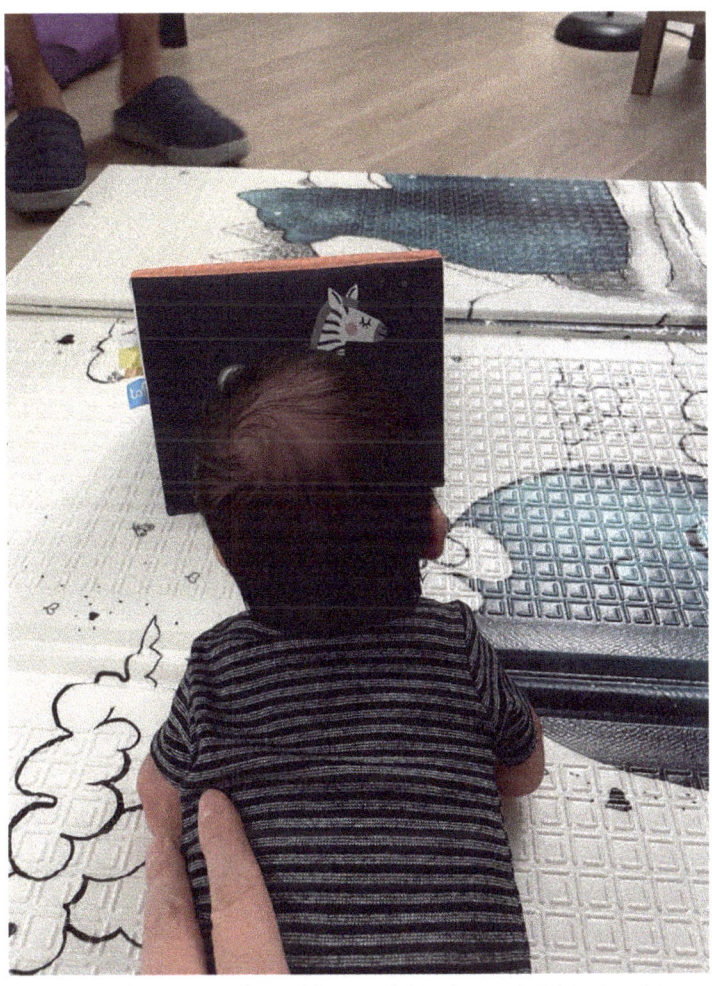

Use your hands at your baby's hips to stabilize them and shift their weight
back. This makes it easier to lift the head.

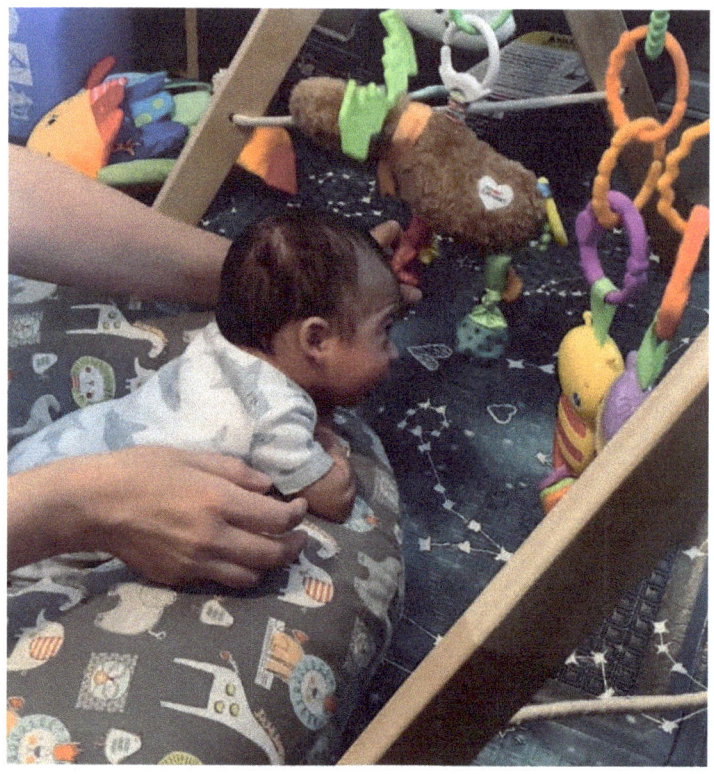

Using a "u" shaped pillow to shift your baby's weight back instead of your hands allows you to call attention to toys, encouraging your baby to look left and right.

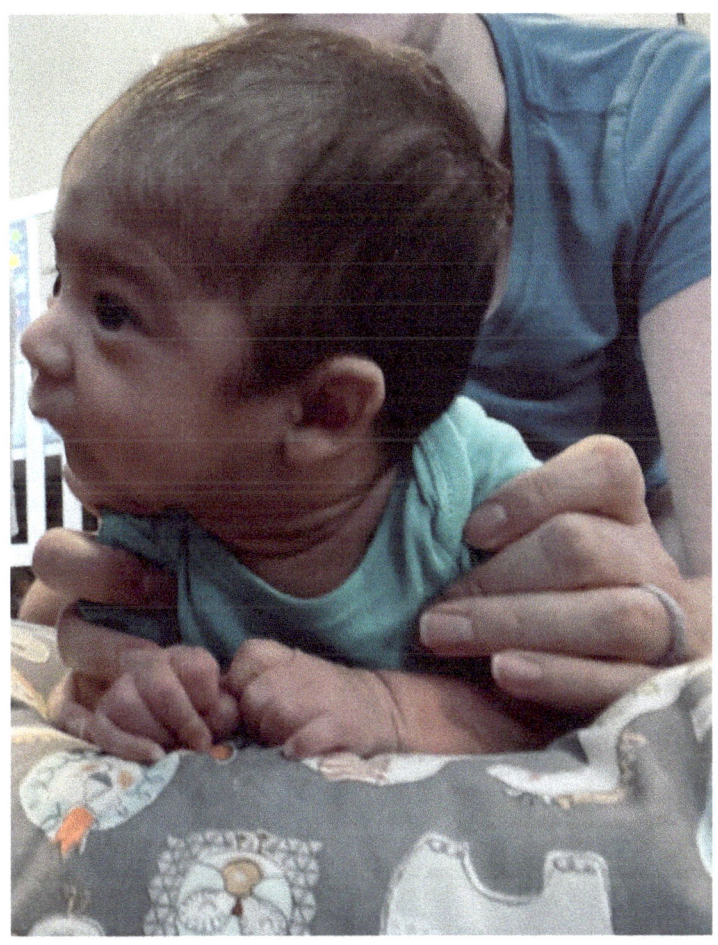

Using a "u" shaped pillow to shift weight back also allows you to provide more support at the shoulders, helping your baby to lift their head higher with more stability.

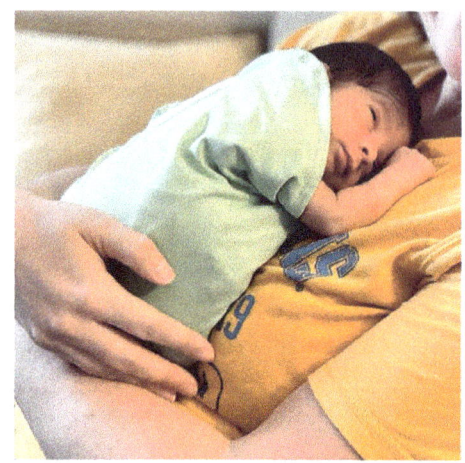

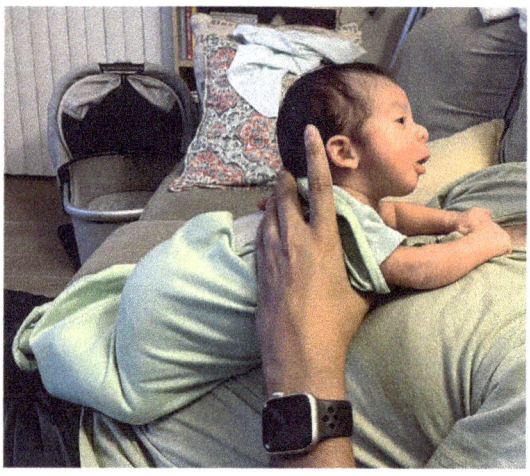

Positioning chest to chest can help babies who don't enjoy tummy time.
Recline back to challenge your baby.

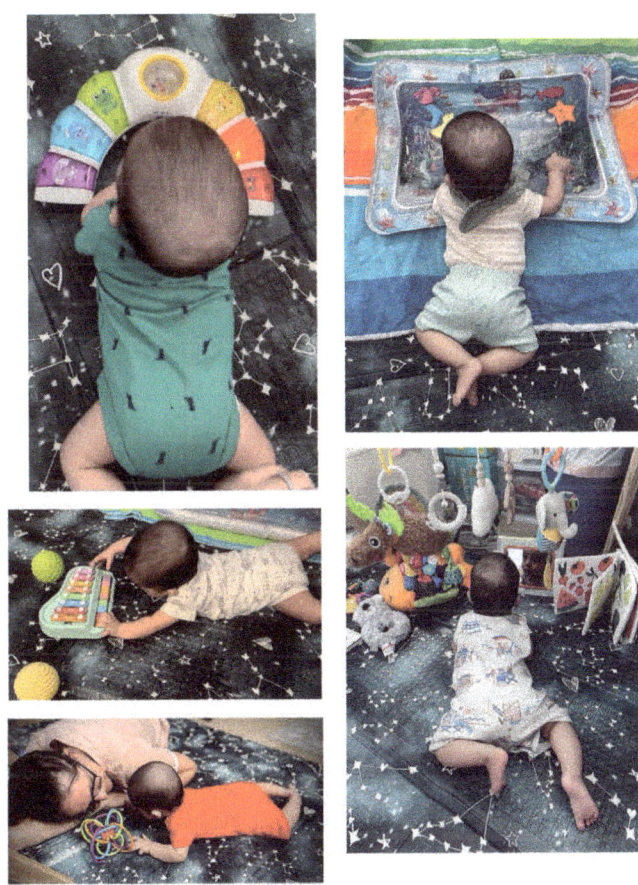

Use colorful and interactive toys such as a light up toy, water mat, mirror, and toy piano to engage your baby and make the position fun. Getting on eye level, making faces and sounds, and playing with your baby help too!

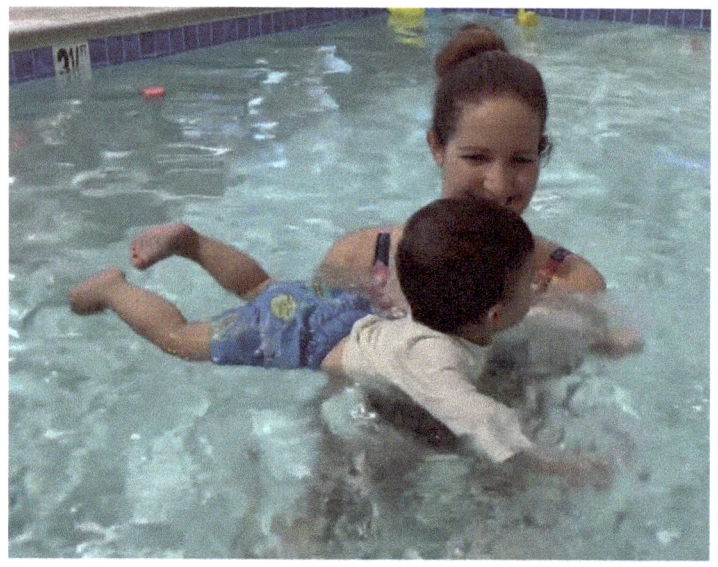

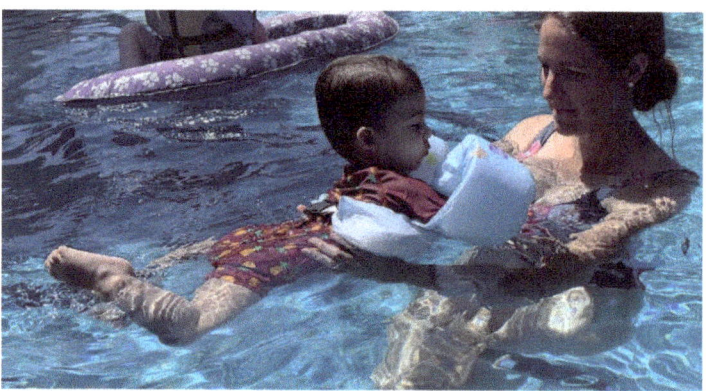

The pool can be another great place to work on tummy time skills. Be sure to observe water safety and consider a "Parent and Me" swimming class.

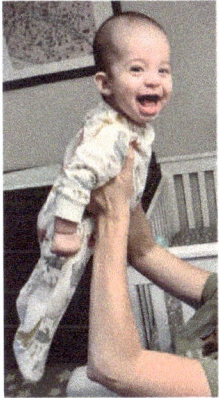

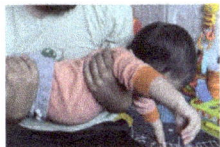

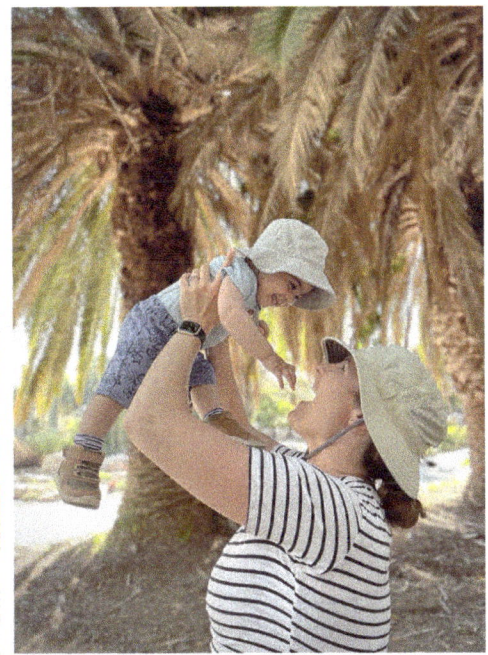

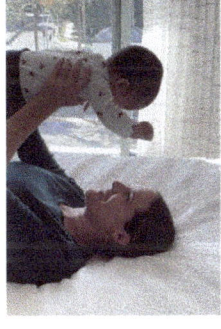

Positioning into "airplane" once your baby has some head control can help further strengthen the neck and back muscles.

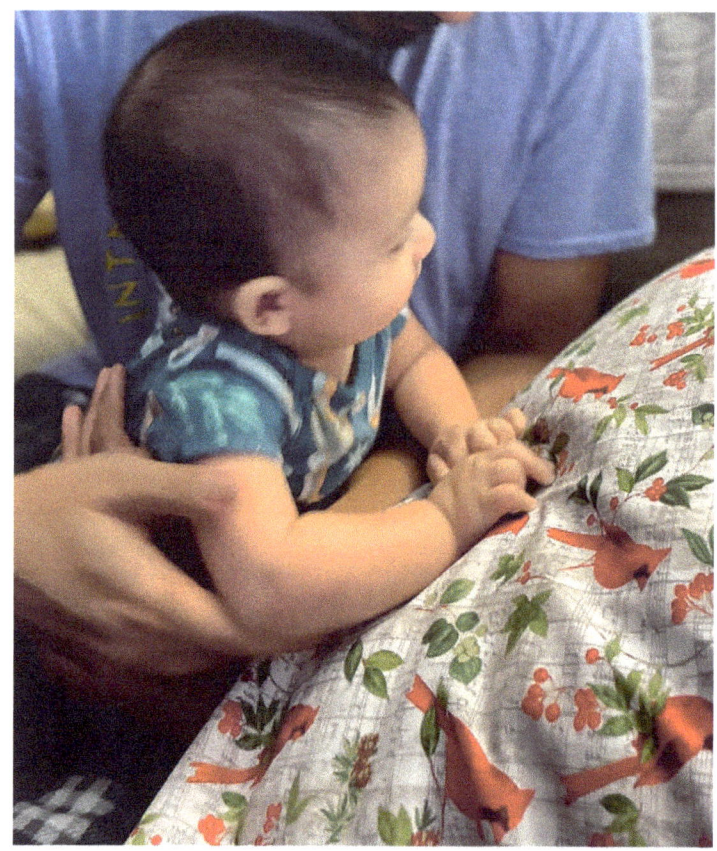

Prop sitting can help strengthen baby's arms and neck while getting weight bearing through the hands. Your baby needs to have head control for this position.

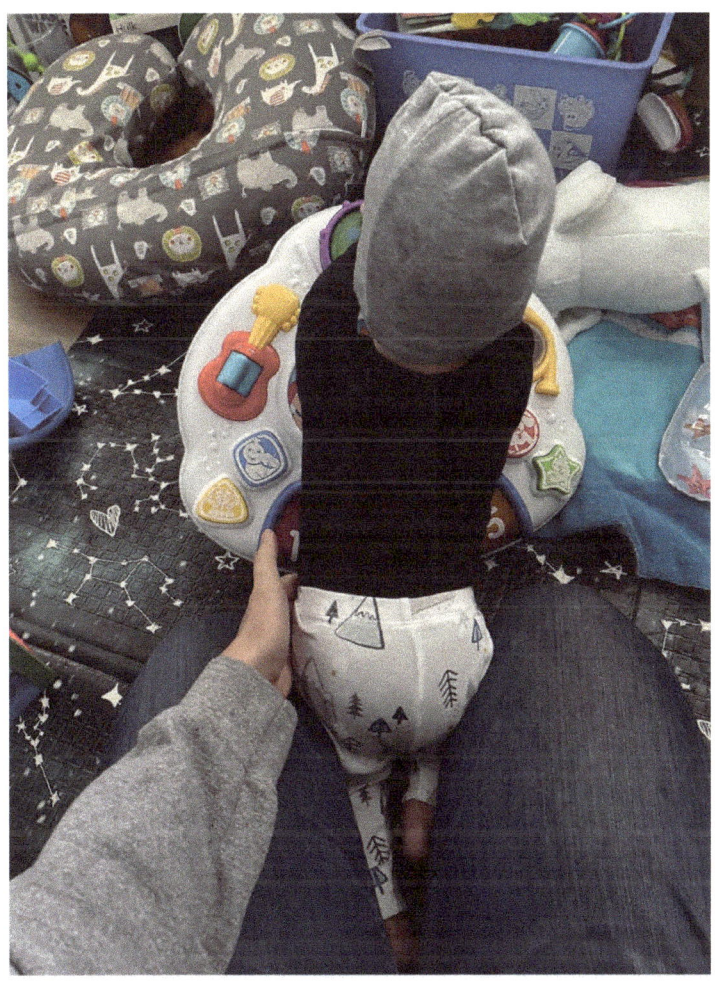

Kneeling with arms on a support surface can also work on strengthening the arms and back of the neck. Again your baby needs head control, and some trunk control. They need to tolerate putting weight through their legs, usually by 7 months old.

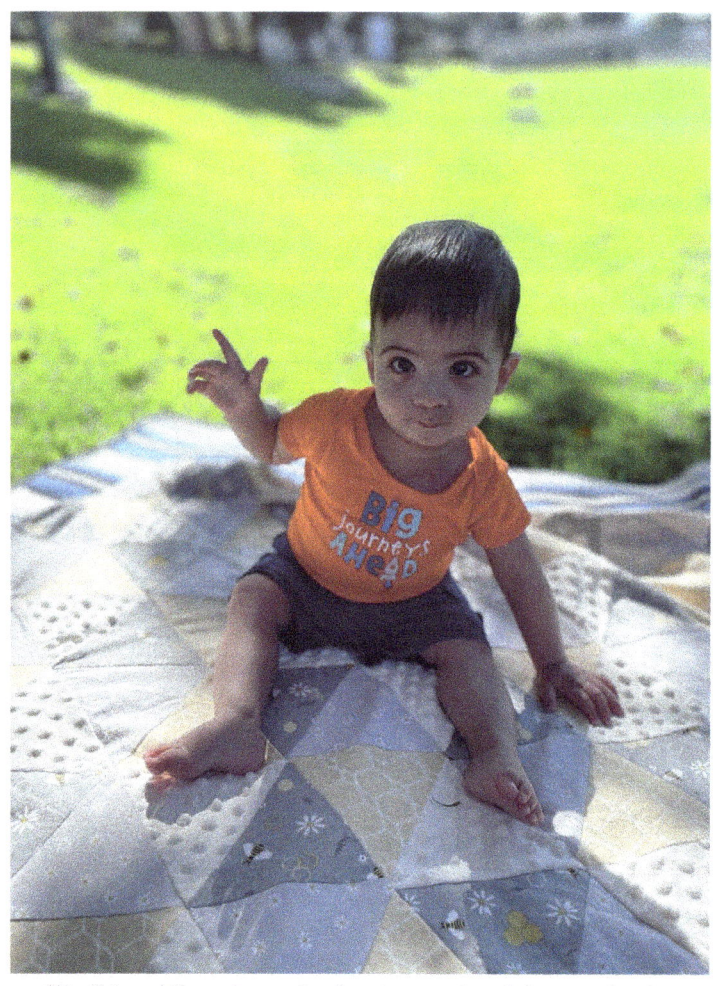

Side sitting while putting one hand on the ground can help strengthen the arms, neck, and core. Your baby should have head control and some trunk control. You can help position your baby by leaning their trunk to one side while reaching to a toy.

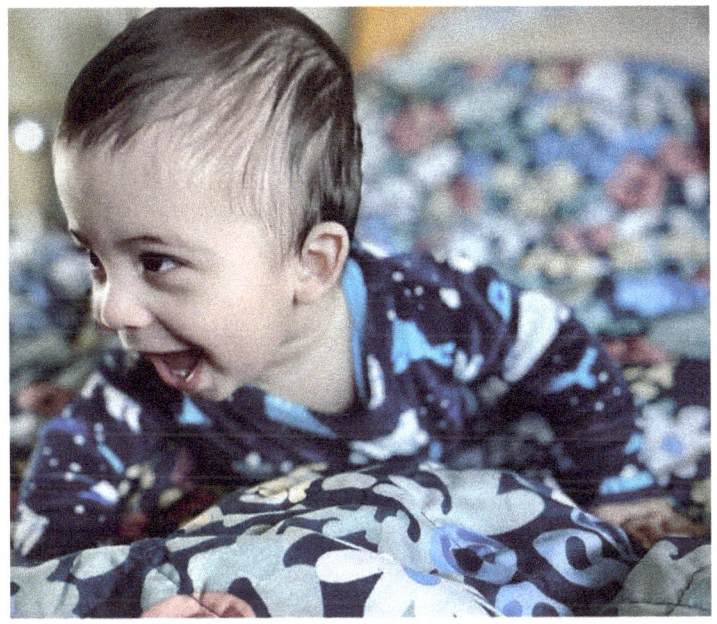

Tummy time champion!

Chapter 3

Rolling

Early independent mobility is one of the most important goals for infants. It's not only for the development of their muscles, but it allows them to start exploring their environment, assisting with cognitive development. Rolling is usually the first form of mobility infants will experience. It is an exciting milestone, but comes with some more challenging diaper changes, and for us, some stress with sleep.

Tummy time and enjoyment in tummy time is one of the keys to accomplishing rolling. If your infant does not like to be on their tummy, they probably won't be trying to roll into that position. It was common for me to see clients who showed potential to roll back to tummy, but they would roll just far enough to get to their toy, then go straight back to their back because they disliked the position so much. Early tummy time with the strategies discussed in the previous chapter are key to preventing this common dilemma.

The other key to rolling is floor time. If your infant spends most of the day contained in your arms, bassinet, swing, or bouncer, they won't have the ability to practice and learn the motor skills required to roll. Rolling to the sides emerges around 3 months old, while back to tummy and tummy to back emerge around 5-6 months old.

To facilitate rolling, start placing toys just out of reach while your baby is doing floor time. You can start by providing some assistance at the hips to roll one leg over the other, then see if your baby will complete the roll by reaching his arm across his body to the toy. Gradually decrease the amount of help you provide to your baby.

Our baby figured out how to roll from his tummy to his back quickly, or so we thought. In reality, he would arch his back because of his reflux and didn't *actually like* being on his tummy. Once his body became bigger, he couldn't roll anymore so he really figured it out closer to 5 months old.

Around 4 months old, our son started liking tummy time, became more engaged with his toys and to our delight rolled to his tummy. It was hard not to just give him the toys. I would wait a minute and let him try to figure out how to get them and I was pleasantly surprised and proud when he managed to do it himself! Sometimes I would step in to prevent him from becoming too frustrated and giving up.

It was exciting to watch him move and explore independently, but diaper changes became more of a challenge! Now that we had to remove the swaddle and he would roll to his tummy to sleep, we experienced many more sleepless nights. It was a bittersweet skill for us.

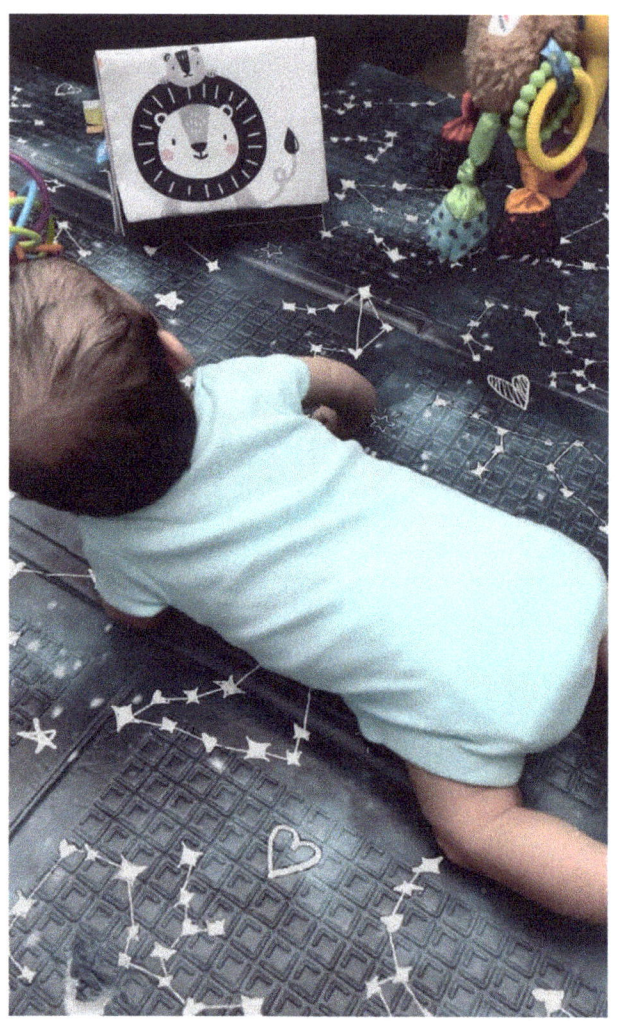

Watch for readiness to roll. Your baby will weight shift completely to one side. It is easier to roll onto the back once the elbow is tucked in past the shoulder.

On Their Own

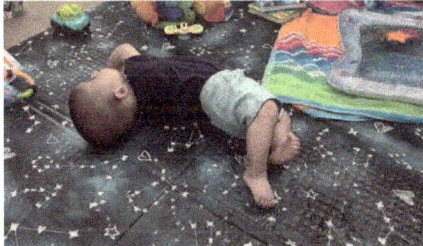

Entice your baby with preferred toys that are just out of reach. They may start by turning their body like this to see the toy.

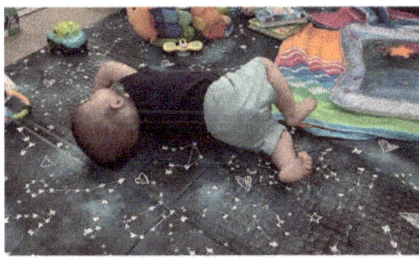

Next, your baby should bring their top leg over the bottom.

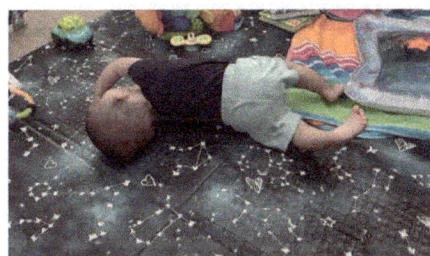

They start extending their top leg and twisting their trunk to complete the roll.

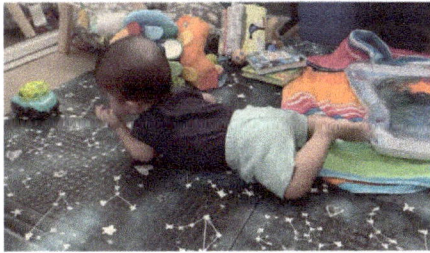

Lastly, your baby will extend the top leg fully as their hand gains support.

With Help

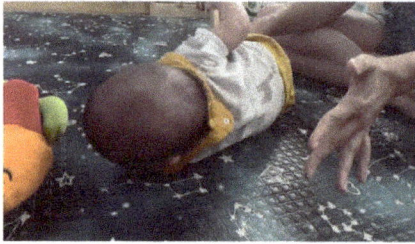

To help your baby roll to their tummy, hold onto the thigh of their top leg as they initiate their roll.

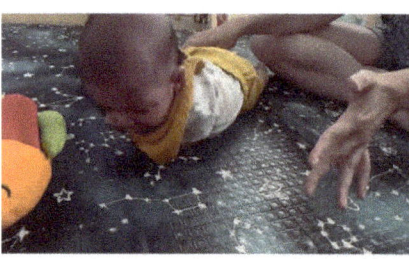

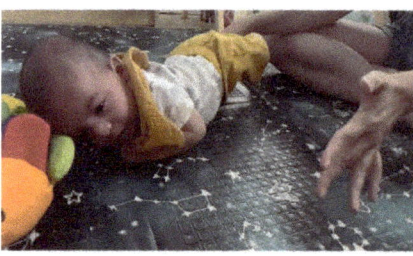

For many babies, the hardest part of the roll is the sidelying to tummy transition. By gently pulling down (toward their toes) on the top thigh, you provide a stretch through the body that helps your baby to lift their head and complete their roll.

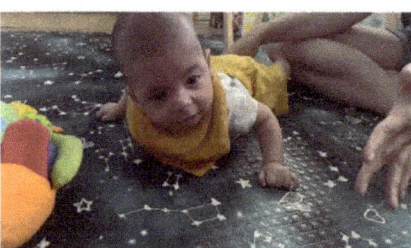

The last piece is clearing the arms so they are not "stuck" under the body. Sometimes babies need help by pulling the same leg. This helps them weight shift to clear their arm.

Chapter 4

Sitting

Acquisition of independent sitting is one of the more exciting skills. It means your baby can sit up and watch things around them and often means you can start introducing solid foods! Plus, babies enjoy being more at eye level with everyone else.

Babies may first learn to "prop" sit by putting weight forward on their hands. This position is cute, but not very functional since they can't use their hands. Prop sitting allows them to observe their environment from a higher vantage point.

Sitting independently emerges around 6 months old, but if your baby is showing good head and trunk control you may be able to put them into a supportive chair sooner. Look for a chair that puts the hips in a neutral or anterior tilt position, as if your baby is sitting on a flat surface or downhill. This position helps your baby to sit with optimal spinal alignment and is preferred over chairs that sling or divot inward, as if sitting on an uphill.

When considering a highchair, look for one that keeps the elbows at about 90 degrees, and has foot support. Ideally, the highchair should be adjustable to accommodate your baby's growth.

When working on independent sitting, it is important to supervise your baby and provide him with a safe place to fall. Sitting may emerge around 6 months, but protective reactions come later. Protective reactions include reaching a hand out to catch yourself when you fall or using your trunk as a counterbalance when reaching too far for a toy.

Play mats are helpful for practicing, but some parents prefer a bed or couch since it has more cushioning. When using a bed or couch, your baby is more at risk of falls from a height. This can be especially harmful and are considered high risk with children who can roll. "U" shaped pillows, are a great alternative because they hug around the hips and provide more extensive cushion with falls sideways or backwards. Protection from forward falls is typically limited so be cautious of the type of toys and surfaces in front of your baby.

I advise my clients to supervise their baby when practicing independent sitting because you can help your baby reach for toys while they simultaneously learn how to safely reposition or catch themselves when they fall. If you want to start supported sitting with supervision earlier hold your baby around their chest while they reach for toys or turn to watch siblings. This engages their core and promotes strengthening of these muscles.

When you notice a position becoming easier for your baby, slowly start introducing challenges. Find the "just right challenge" for your child. For example, maybe your child has become very good at sitting with only some support at their hips. You can make it harder by encouraging your baby to reach outside of their base of support while still providing support at the hips. This challenges their balance and requires them to use their core muscles to re-center themselves. You can also remove your support from the hips and just hover, ready to catch your baby as they focus on an unmoving object, like a light up toy or mirror.

If your baby is good at sitting and reaching, you can progress them to side sitting with one arm down, reaching even further away towards a toy. You can further challenge their core strength and balance by sitting them on your lap or on a chair without foot support and have them reach to a toy or bouncing them. This forces them to shift their weight around and use their core to get back to the starting position. There are so many fun ways to strengthen your baby in sitting!

One position to avoid is "w" sitting. This is when your baby sits in a kneeling position, but their feet are out wider than their knees. This puts their knees closer together and their legs look like a "w". Kneeling is a great position to practice strengthening, as discussed elsewhere in this book. Kneeling should be done with feet together, under the baby's hips. When you see your baby "w" sitting, try to reposition them with their legs in front of their body, side sitting, or kneeling. "W" sitting is common, but frequent positioning can put stress on the knees and hips. It is thought to be a result of decreased core strength, as the position gives children a wider base of support to balance while sitting.

Our experience with sitting was much easier compared to tummy time. Our baby loved being upright, looking around our home, watching our cat, and reaching for the toys too high to reach from his tummy.

As a transition between supported sitting to independent sitting, we made a small "desk" for him using diaper boxes. We made the cardboard edges smooth and supervised him while he used his "desk". We found this helpful because he sat up taller trying to reach his toys. We would couple this with reaching his toys hanging from his "gym" while supporting his hips.

Our baby sat for brief periods around 6 months, but we kept a close eye on him until he mastered catching himself when he lost his balance, which happened closer to 8-9 months old. As his sitting became more advanced, we switched from a bassinet stroller to an upright stroller and he loved being able to see more on our walks! This was one of our favorite time periods as parents.

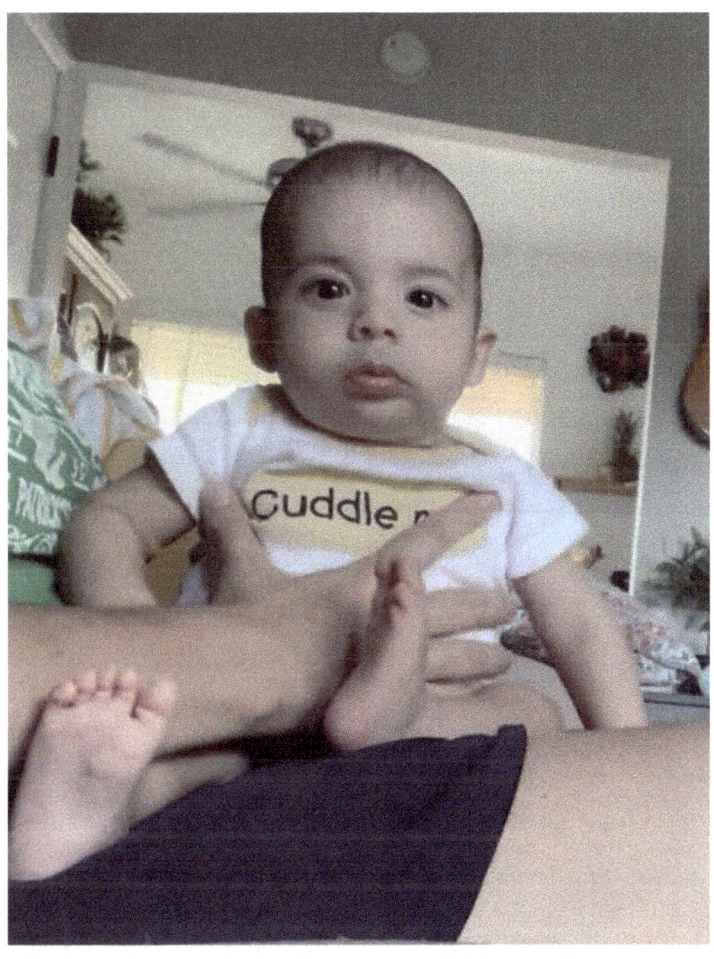

Start by having your baby sit with support around their chest. They must have head control for this position.

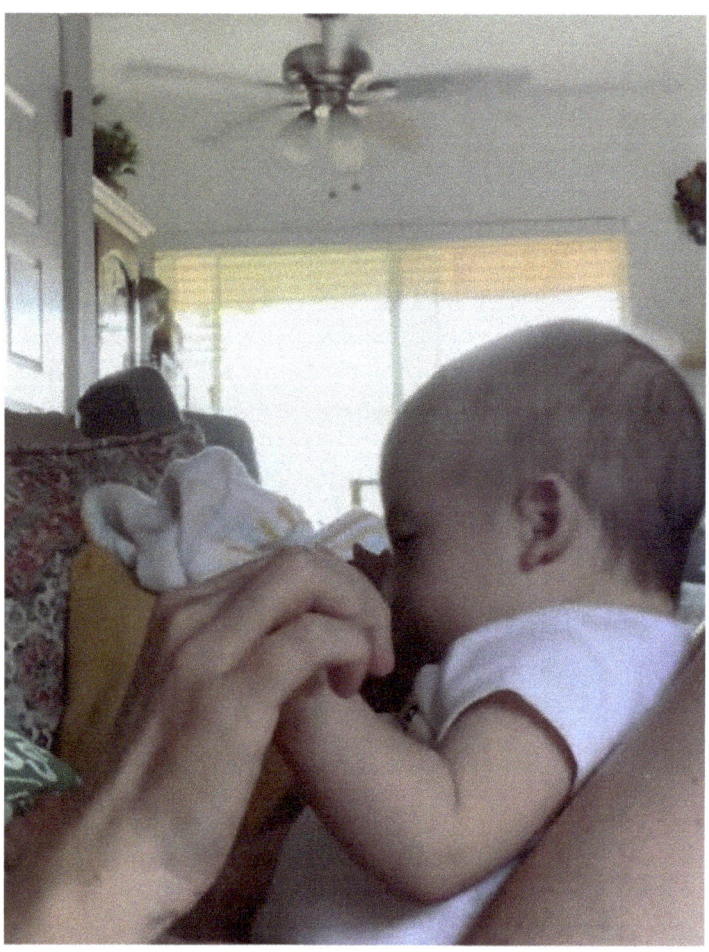

You can have your baby practice strengthening their neck, core, and arms by pulling themselves up to sit from a reclined position on your legs. Your baby should initiate the movement. Your hands are just their support.

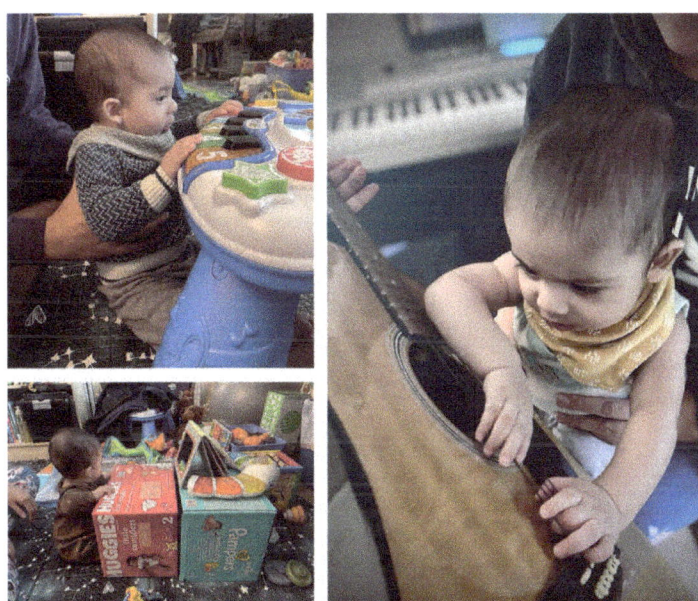

Have your baby work on strengthening their back and shoulder muscles by reaching up to toys at shoulder height.

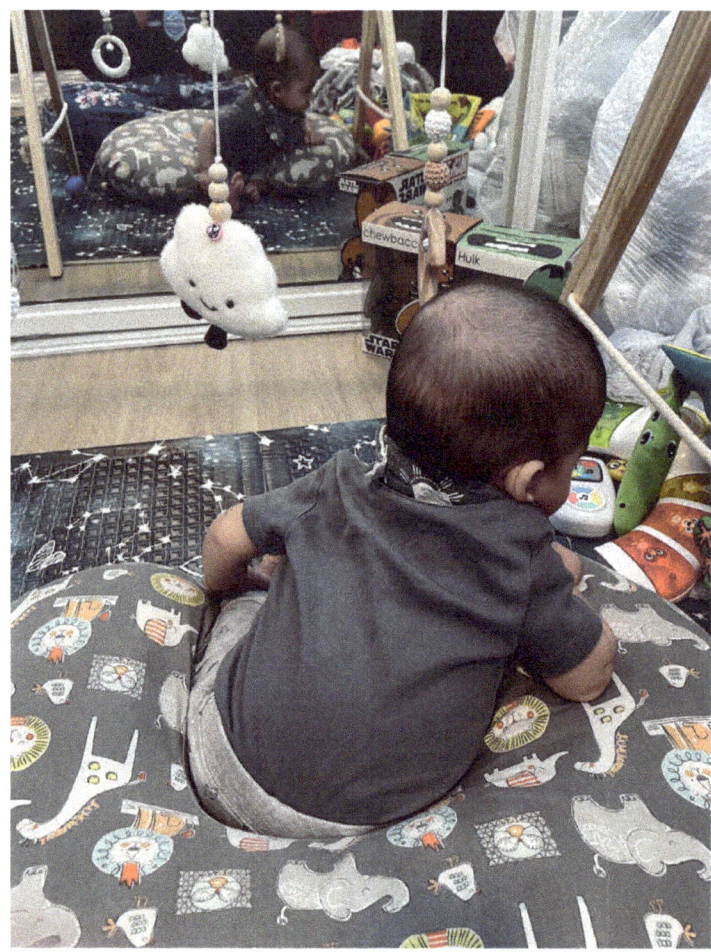

Using a "u" shaped pillow around the hips can help your baby start practicing some independent sitting earlier on. Your baby can catch themselves using the pillow and work on repositioning themselves upright. Your baby must have head control and emerging trunk control for this position.

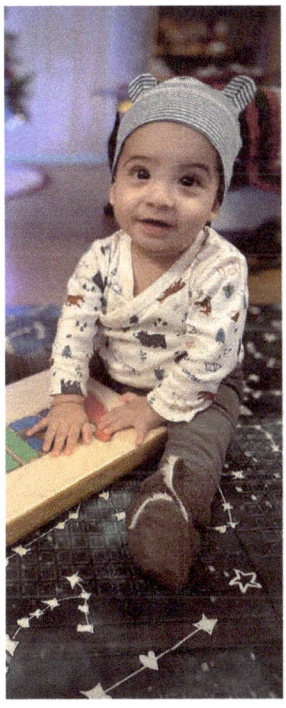
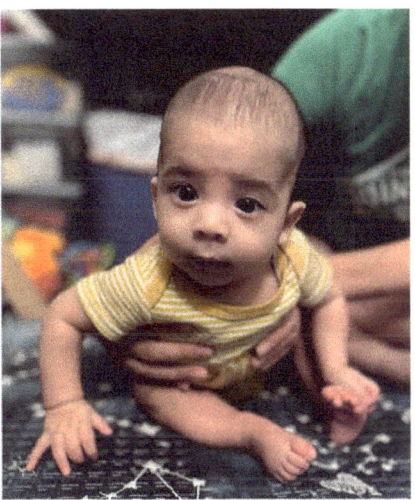

Prop sitting might be the first independent sitting position for your baby. It can be useful to practice weight bearing through the arms and strengthening the back and neck.

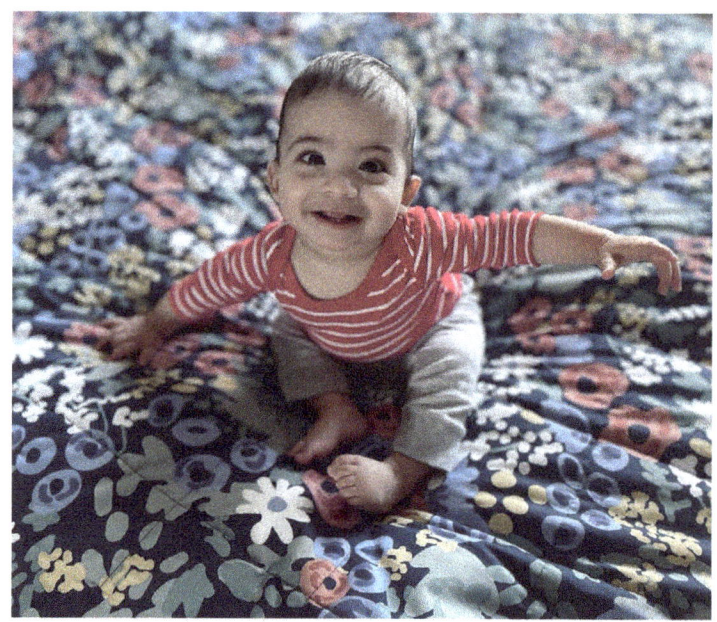

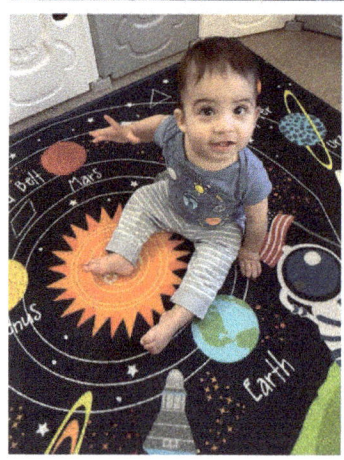

As your baby masters sitting, you can have them reach for a toy further away by putting one hand down to strengthen their core, arms, and head.

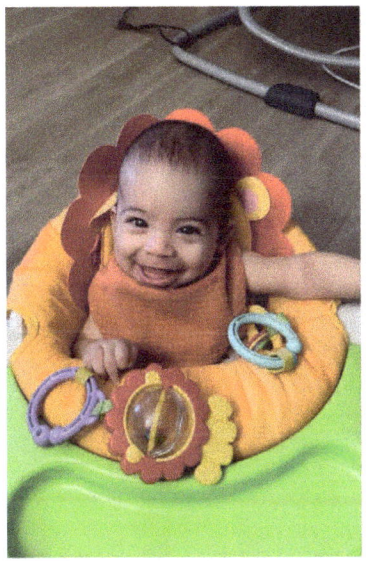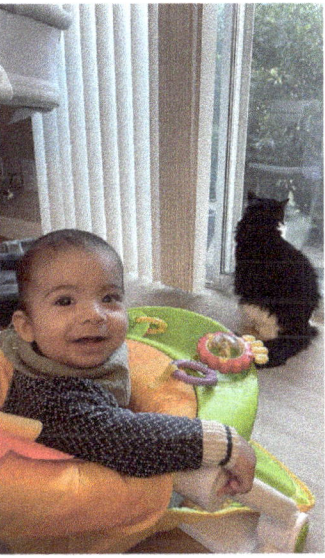

Look for a chair that positions the hips in a downward or flat position (like sitting downhill). Your baby must have head control and some trunk control for this position.

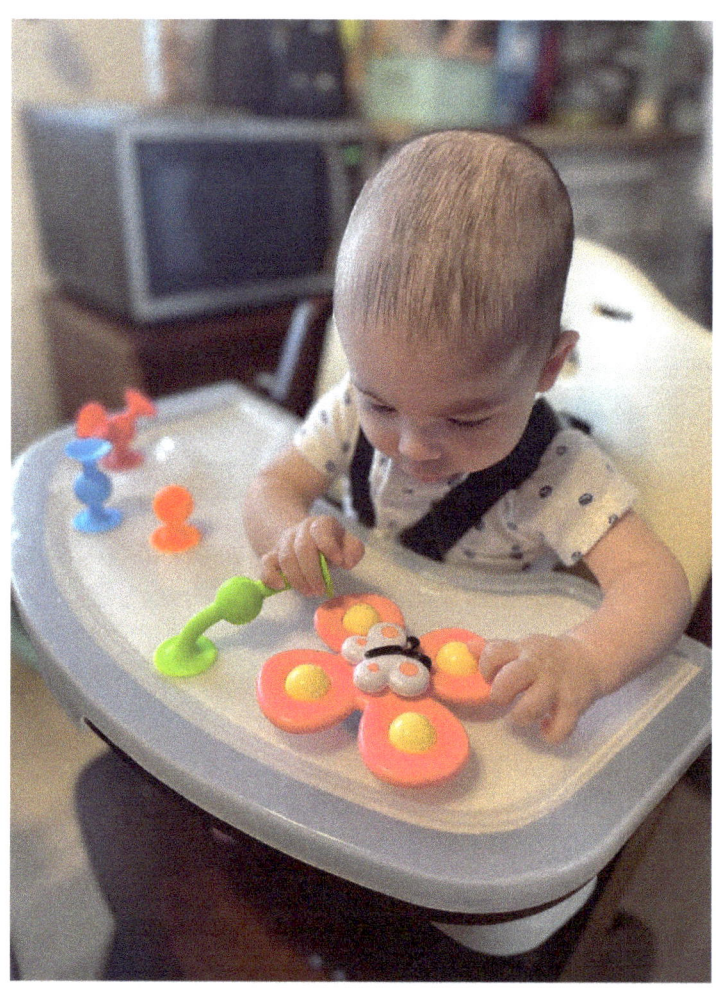

Look for highchairs that place your baby's elbows at 90 degrees and allows their feet to be flat on a support. Your baby must have head control and some trunk control.

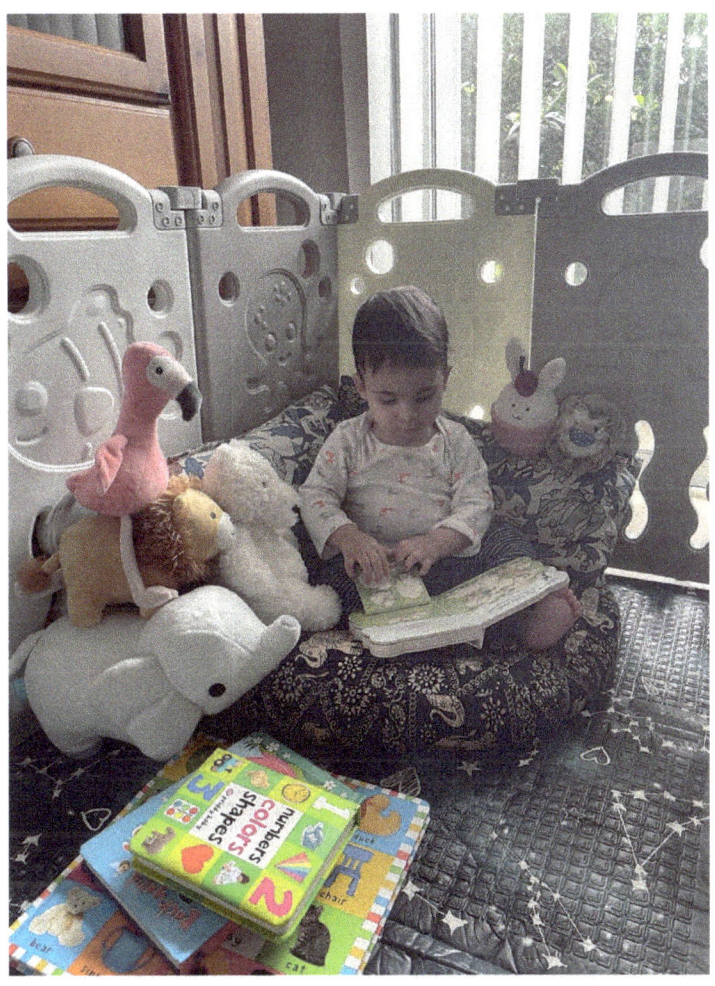

Even after your baby has mastered sitting, be sure they have a safe space to
fall. It will take them a while to also master their protective reactions, which
help them correct a loss of balance.

Chapter 5

Crawling

Crawling is usually the first form of forward mobility your child will achieve. Although, the need for children to achieve crawling has been challenged in recent years, it is an excellent form of exercise to strengthen the abdominal and upper extremity muscles and build coordination. Recently, the CDC removed it as a necessary motor milestone, which has been controversial for many physical therapists. Current research supports the acquisition of early independent mobility, regardless of how that mobility is achieved. However, there has not been sufficient research to support the need to specifically achieve crawling.

Physical therapists have theorized that crawling is an important skill to facilitate the development of visual depth perception, progress bilateral coordination, and possibly decrease incidence of pain and postural impairments later in life.

Contrary to these theories, many families will recall how their sons and daughters "skipped" crawling without any noted deficits. Some children will crawl in different ways such as butt scooting, asymmetrical crawling, or "army" crawling on the belly. In certain cultures, crawling is not encouraged for a variety of reasons including possible safety of the living environment.

Personally, I think crawling is an important milestone to strive for but give your child grace if they are progressing faster with their standing and walking skills. Crawling is a good precursor to climbing over obstacles at home and on the playground, and it's a great way to strengthen and build coordination.

To encourage crawling, start with your baby in tummy time. Work on reaching for a toy, encouraging your child to alternate arms. As your child is becoming stronger and it appears easier for them to shift their weight, position toys or another motivator just out of their reach. Make it close enough that it is "achievable" but far enough away that they need to move their body to get there. Many infants will start with "army crawling", where they pull themselves mostly with their arms, then progress to hands and knees crawling.

To help your child progress with hands and knees crawling, start with kneeling and hands and knees play. Kneeling allows your child to work on strengthening the hip muscles that will help push off. You can also use kneeling to promote weightbearing through the hands, which is easier than pushing up on flat ground. For example, it's more difficult doing push-ups flat on the ground compared to doing a wall push-up. A kneeling position makes the task easier for children having trouble with tummy time. Kneeling is easily performed with a couch arm rest or a toy that is inclined.

Hands and knees positioning can be obtained over your leg, a "u" shaped pillow, or a large towel roll. You can then have your child work on reaching for a toy or playing with a toy in this position. Sometimes you will need to help your baby keep their hips and knees flexed if they're having trouble using their abdominal muscles.

Once we figured out how to make tummy time easier and more enjoyable, our son achieved crawling without much intervention from us. One day, he just started pulling himself toward a toy that was out of his reach. It was such an exciting moment, followed by the realization that we needed to finish baby proofing as soon as possible! He was about 8 months old when he started army crawling and about 9 months for hands and knees. I practiced physical therapy exercises that I typically prescribe to my clients with him, but really he did most of the work on his own. This was the end of sitting still for long periods when we went out, but it was very much worth it!

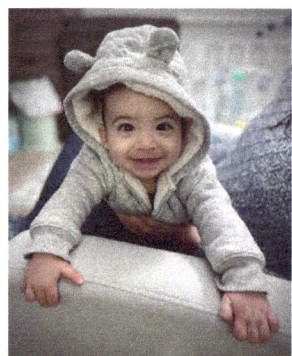

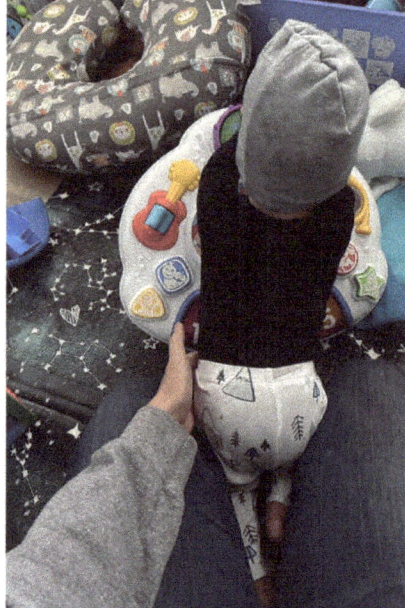

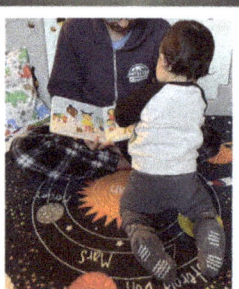

Kneeling at a couch or chair armrest to allow weight bearing through the arms and knees strengthens the hips, arms, core, and neck muscles for crawling. You can have your baby reach to toys or faces to advance the position.

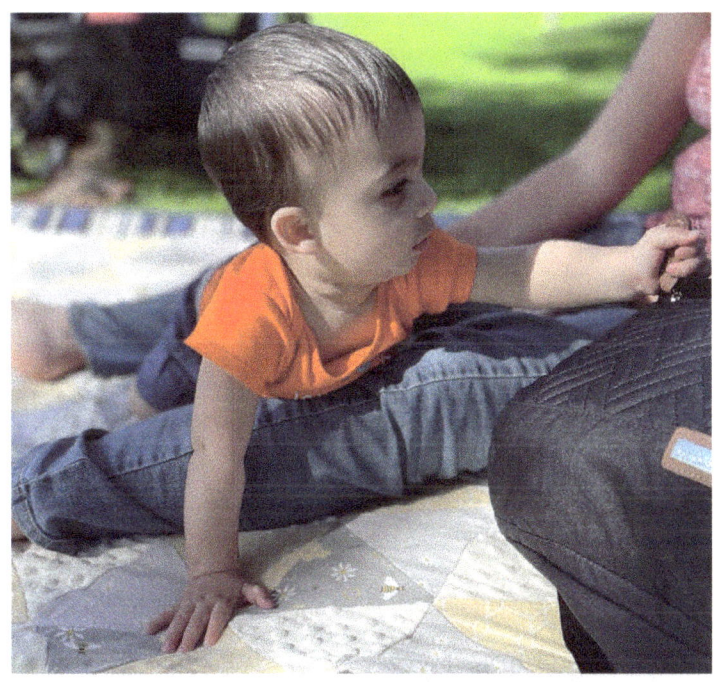

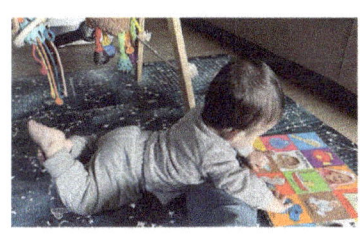 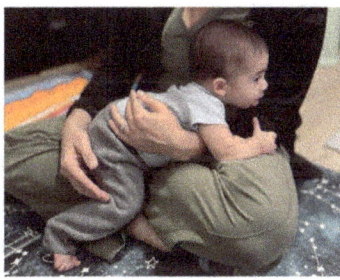

Positioning in hands and knees over your leg is another way to work toward crawling. Have your baby reach to objects to advance the position.

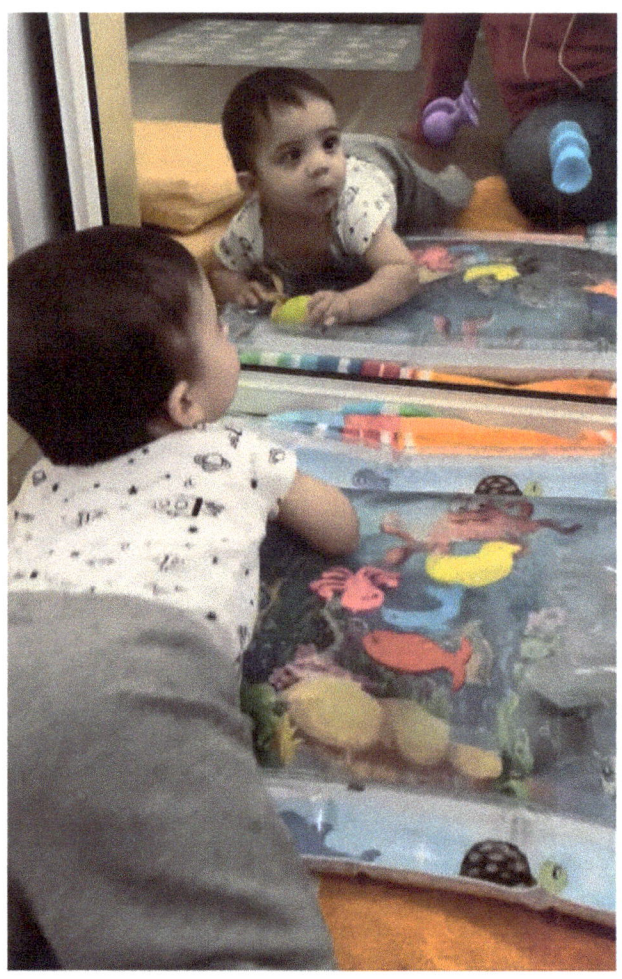

Once your baby shows strength in the hands and knees position, place toys just out of reach to encourage moving forward. Your baby might start with "army crawling" first.

Chapter 6

Standing

Standing is one of the biggest precursors to walking. Your child is up, can see the world at a new level and is ready to explore. Independent standing usually emerges around 10 months old, but your child may stand with support or stand while holding onto furniture before this time. Usually, I don't encourage practicing standing until at least 7 months of age to allow adequate core and hip strength to develop, preventing inappropriate stresses to the legs.

Some kids take longer to master standing for a variety of reasons including larger head size, larger body size, smaller feet, pronated or flat feet, among many others. Standing is about mastering stability and balance. For kids with a larger head size, balancing the heavier top half of their body is tricky in standing. Larger body size requires increased strength to support standing. Smaller feet mean a smaller base of support to balance on, if the body size is not proportional. Flat feet are normal for infants, but when they are exceedingly pronated it can change the center of gravity, narrow the base of support, and make balancing more difficult. Most of these qualities are not concerning and although your child might stand and walk later than peers, it should not impact their motor skills in the long run.

Before discussing how to encourage standing, I want to address walkers. I am talking about the walkers your baby sits in and uses their feet to move forward and backwards, not the push toys that your baby needs to be able to stand on their own to use. Baby walkers are very popular for a variety of reasons. They're cute, readily available, and appear to give your baby early strengthening for the legs. Additionally, for busy parents it gives you a place to put your baby while you tend to other responsibilities.

Unfortunately, walkers are not recommended by pediatricians or physical therapists because they are a safety risk. Baby walkers commonly cause preventable falls and are especially dangerous in households with stairs. Additionally, babies can reach higher surfaces when sitting in these walkers leading to an increased number of burns and poisoning accidents. Lastly, babies using baby walkers can easily get to unsupervised locations such as pools and bathtubs increasing the risk of drownings. There are safety warnings for baby walkers, but they are still widely sold in the United States.

There are additional concerns about the extra forces and pressures on the hips and knees when kids are not developmentally ready, the alignment of the hips in the devices, and the risk of developing "toe walking" later on (it is easy to propel the walker using solely the toes rather than other muscles of the legs).

To encourage standing, start by placing toys and preferred items up on a higher surface. Cognition drives motor learning! If there isn't a reason for your baby to get into standing, they aren't as likely to do it. Make sure your set-up is safe, surrounded by safe areas to fall including plenty of corner protectors. Your little one's balance is going to take time to develop, and practice makes perfect, which means falls are expected!

Take opportunities to encourage standing while your baby is watching other older kiddos. If your child doesn't have a sibling, cousins, or friend's kids readily available; then your local playground or kid friendly space may work. Watching other kids standing and walking helps with motor learning and motivation. When you're out, let your child practice standing in your lap to see higher over a table or across the room. Point out something they can see from their new vantage point.

As you practice on the floor, you can slowly remove your support as you feel your baby get more stable. Keep your hands close though! As mentioned before, falling is an expected and important part of development, but should be made safe and injury-free.

When our son was really working toward standing and walking, we started spending a lot of time at our local park. The playground there was popular with toddlers and he enjoyed watching them. We would have picnics in the grass nearby and just let him observe. He would practice standing using us or the stroller for support. I feel he really progressed with his upright stability and mobility from these exposures.

We also used a large baby gate to create a play yard at home, which had multiple places for him to pull himself up into standing. He was able to stand by himself for brief periods of time around 10 months of age.

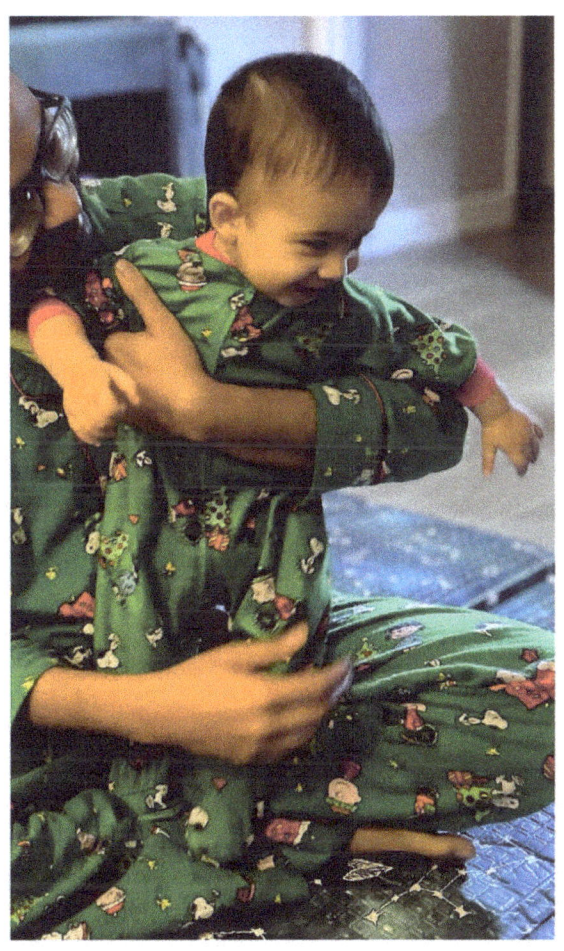

Holding your baby at the chest and hips can help them feel and be more stable in supported standing. This allows them to practice weight bearing through their feet with less demand on their core muscles.

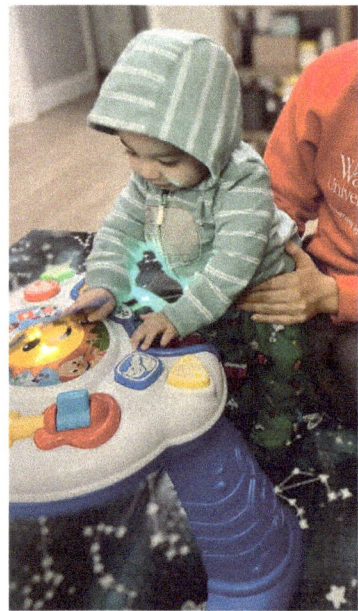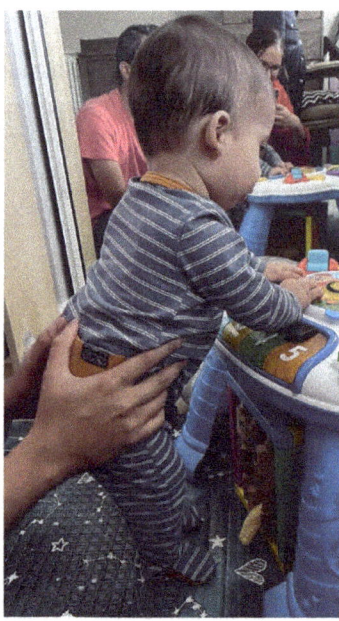

Practice standing at a support surface. Use your hands at the hips to provide support. If your baby likes to position on their toes persistently, use your hands to push down on their hips, shifting their weight to their heels and providing more pressure through the whole foot. Intermittently going on the toes is normal and important to develop the calf muscles.

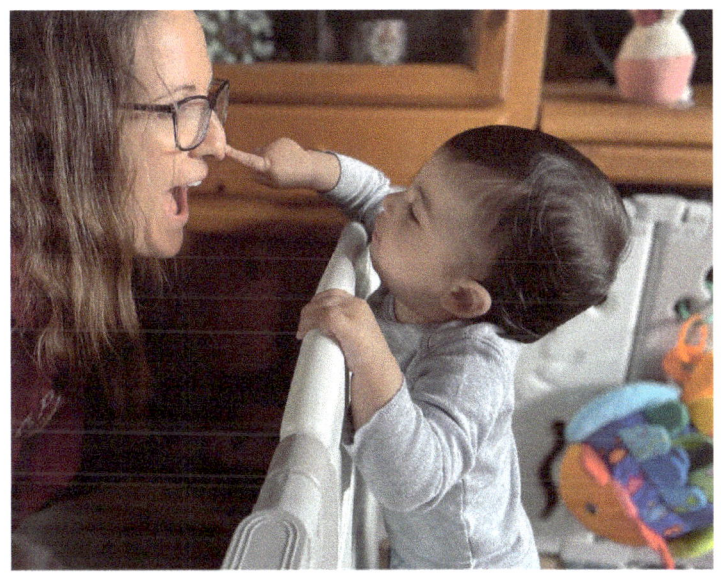

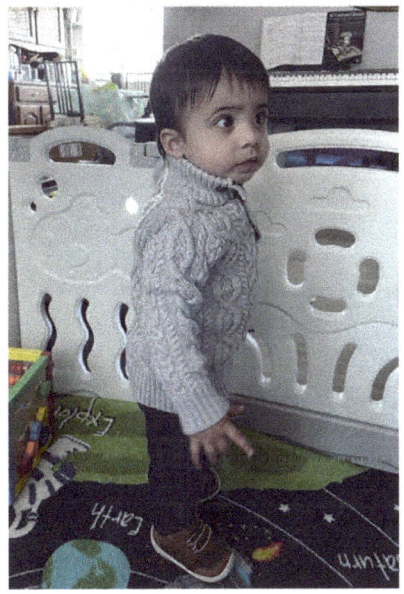

As your baby becomes more confident standing at a stable support surface, encourage them to let go with one hand to challenge their balance.

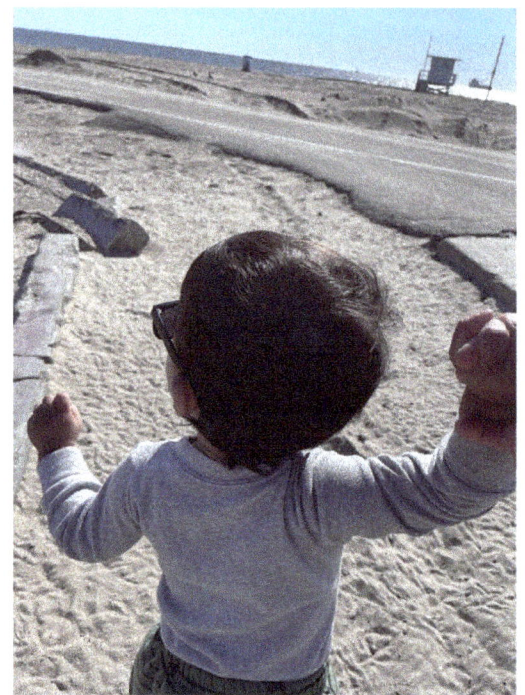

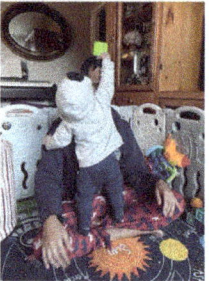

Practice standing with support on uneven surfaces.
Uneven surfaces can be legs, pillows, grass, and sand,
among other options.

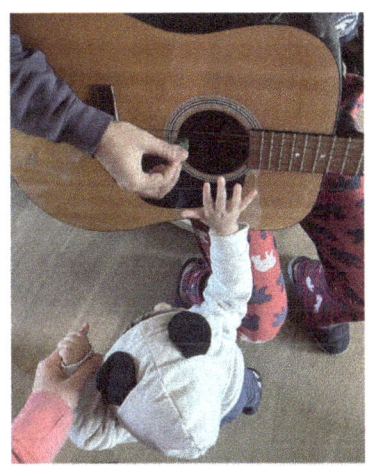

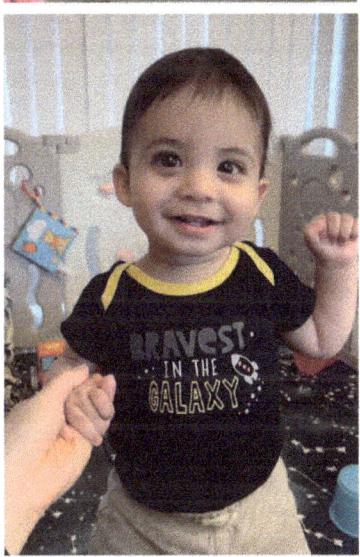

Gradually decrease your support as your baby becomes stronger in standing, moving from 2 hands held to 1 hand held. Encourage them to reach up or to the sides to challenge their balance.

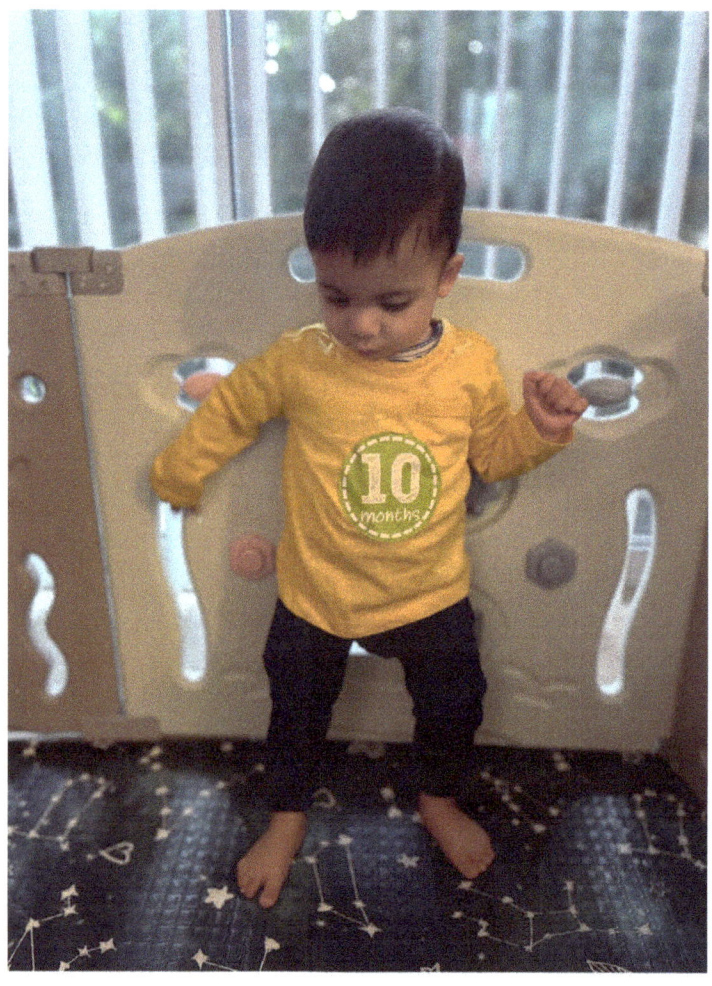

Build your baby's confidence with standing by having them stand with their back against a wall or steady support.

Chapter 7

Walking

Finally, we have arrived at walking! In my career, this is the skill every parent was striving for and for good reason. Walking means your child has more freedom, can explore their world at a new level, and keep up with their peers. Independent walking usually occurs between 12-15 months of age. Fortunately, most children will achieve walking without much intervention from their parents. But here are some tips on how to encourage the progression to independent walking.

First, let me discuss shoes. Shoe wear, and lack thereof, is an important consideration when your child is progressing to walking. Shoes are important to protect your child's feet from injuries, such as stepping on a sharp object, and shielding them from weather.

Despite this, allowing time to be barefoot is crucial. Being barefoot facilitates strengthening of the small muscles of the feet and has been found to help with arch formation. Barefoot feet are also exposed to a variety of textures, which helps with sensory development.

Usually, I recommend a combination of time being barefoot and time in shoes. Shoe wear might best be done when outside in areas where injury may occur, such as in the presence of hot asphalt or potentially sharp twigs. Barefoot practice might be facilitated in the home, on grass, or in the sand.

When teaching your child to walk on their own, start small and focus on building their confidence. In my experience, only some children would try bouts of walking before they were fully confident they could do so without falling. When parents would "back up" to see if they would go further, often their confidence would waiver and they would lose trust in walking to their parents, especially if they fell in the process.

Begin by slowly decreasing support, starting with encouraging cruising holding onto the couch, playpen, or table, then walking with 2 hands held, then 1 hand held, then taking a few steps between supports, and finally walking a few feet. Once your child walks with hands held, you can incorporate walking over uneven surfaces to challenge their balance and strengthen their legs. As mentioned previously, going to a local park to watch other kids can assist with motor learning and motivation for your child. Be aware of your own posture when bending to help your baby. If you're experiencing back pain, it may be time for your own physical therapy!

The first steps our son took were right before his first birthday, just 2 steps. He saved the longest walk for his birthday, when he walked about 10 feet from my husband to me. It was the best birthday treat!

We noticed he would walk on his toes, which is normal when done intermittently up until 2 years old. It is an important way for babies to strengthen their calves for jumping and running. Our son went on his toes frequently, so we put him in high top supportive shoes when we went out and let him be barefoot at home. He no longer walks on his toes and his foot arches have developed well.

Walking meant a new level of baby proofing. As our son became faster and could walk longer distances, keeping him safe became good exercise for us!

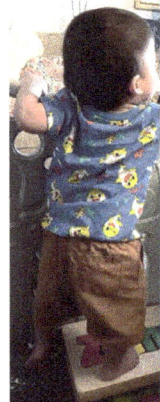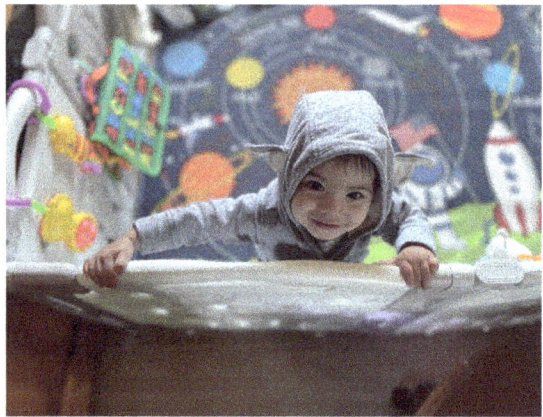

Cruising is a great way for your baby to progress their walking. Use uneven surfaces or steps to challenge their balance and strengthen their ankles, legs, and core muscles.

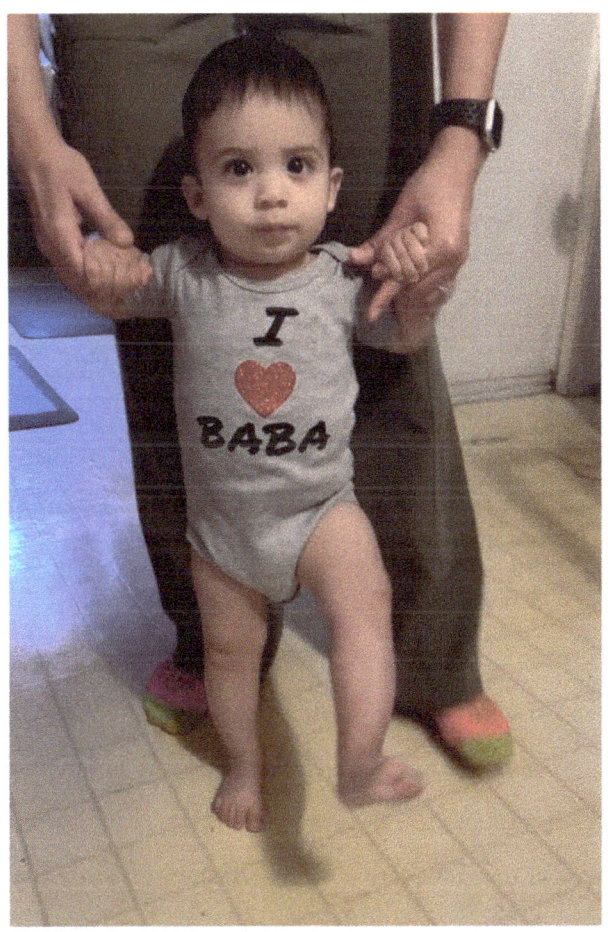

Start walking with 2 hands held. You can help shift your baby's weight side to side by guiding with your hands. Try to keep your baby's hands lower down to their sides to encourage more natural movement.

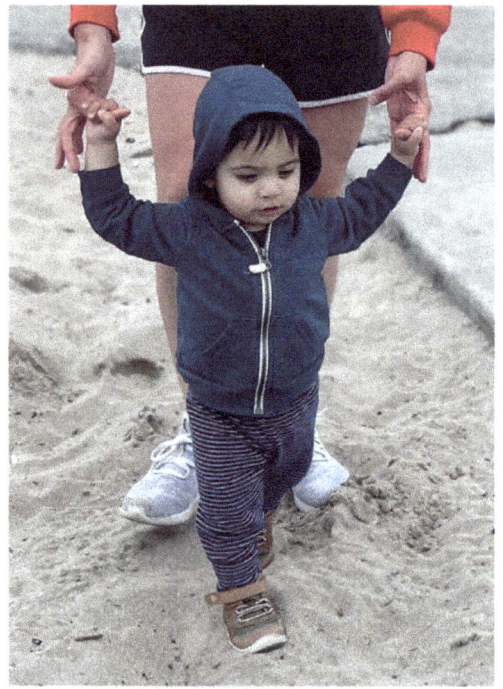

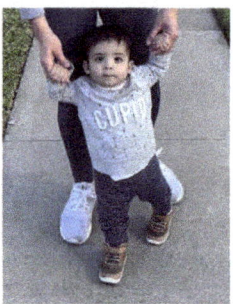

Progressing walking on different surfaces. We preferred wearing shoes outdoors and practiced walking barefoot indoors. These high top supportive shoes also helped addressed some persistent tendency toward toe walking.

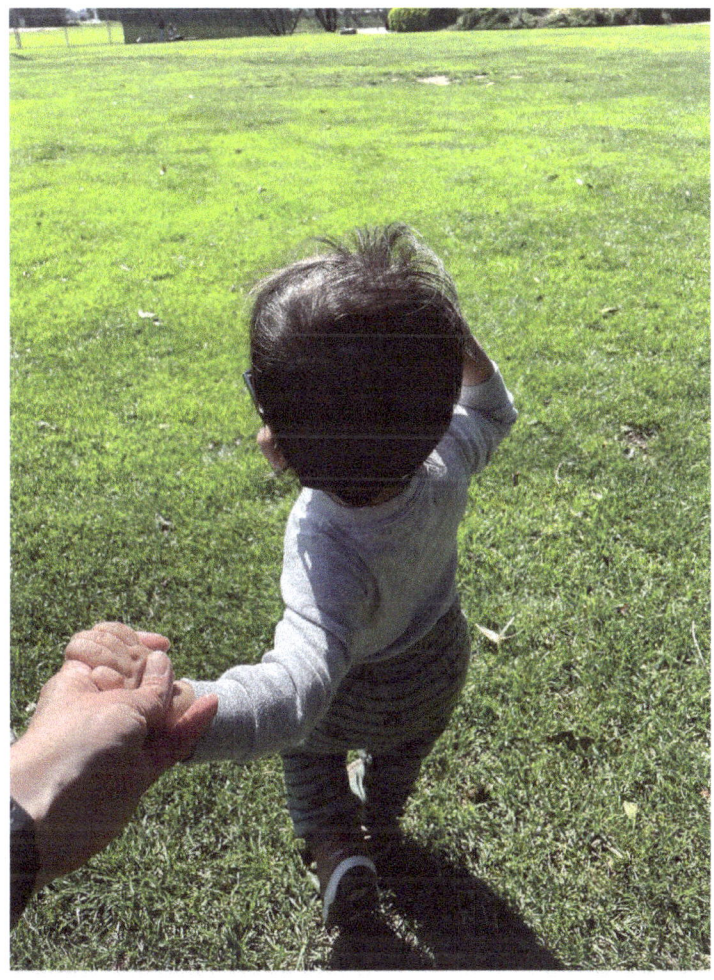

Gradually decrease support to 1 hand as you notice your baby gaining more balance and trunk control. Sometimes giving your baby something to hold in the free hand will help their focus, such as a toy.

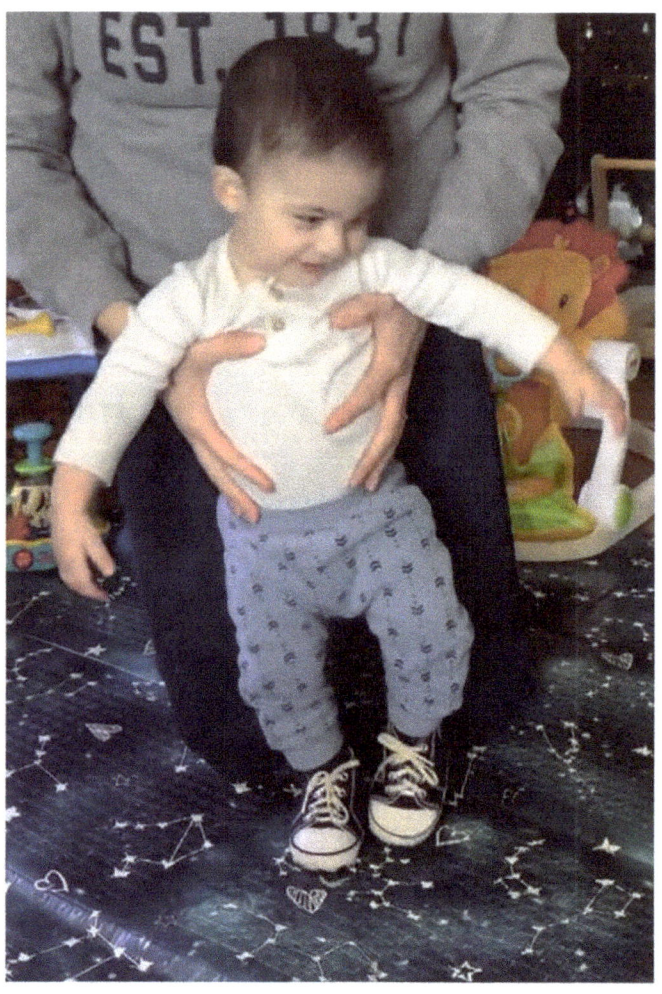

Positioning your hands at your baby's tummy with fingers pointed down to the toes can help you better facilitate weight shifting to progress independent leg advancement.

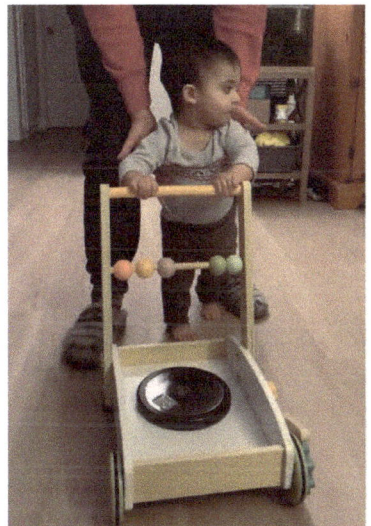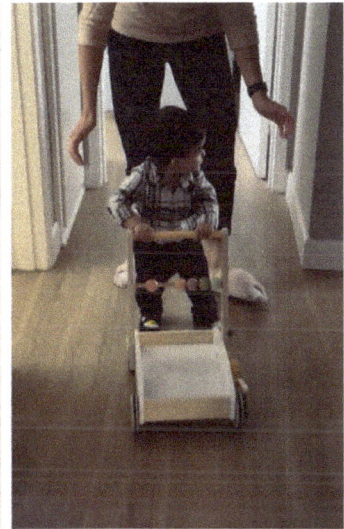

Using a push toy can build confidence and independence with walking. Sometimes putting a weight or providing resistance will make it easier to control for your baby. Stay close by when practicing walking, even with a push toy support.

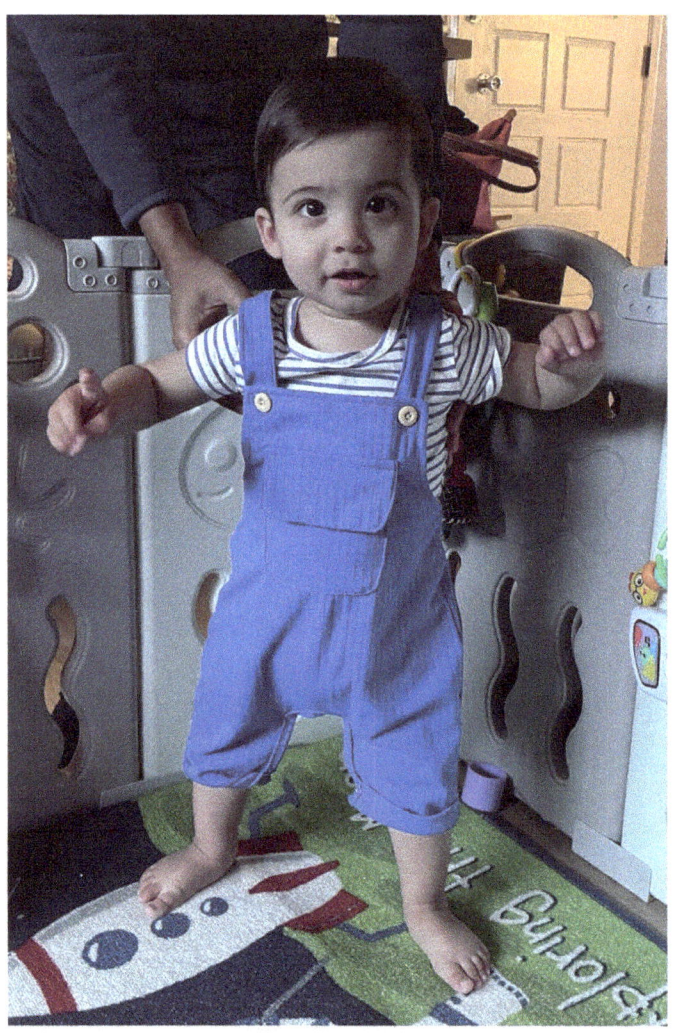

If your baby seems ready to walk but still clings nervously to your hand, you can practice walking while holding onto their shoulders or upper clothing. This way they feel more secure without truly using your support.

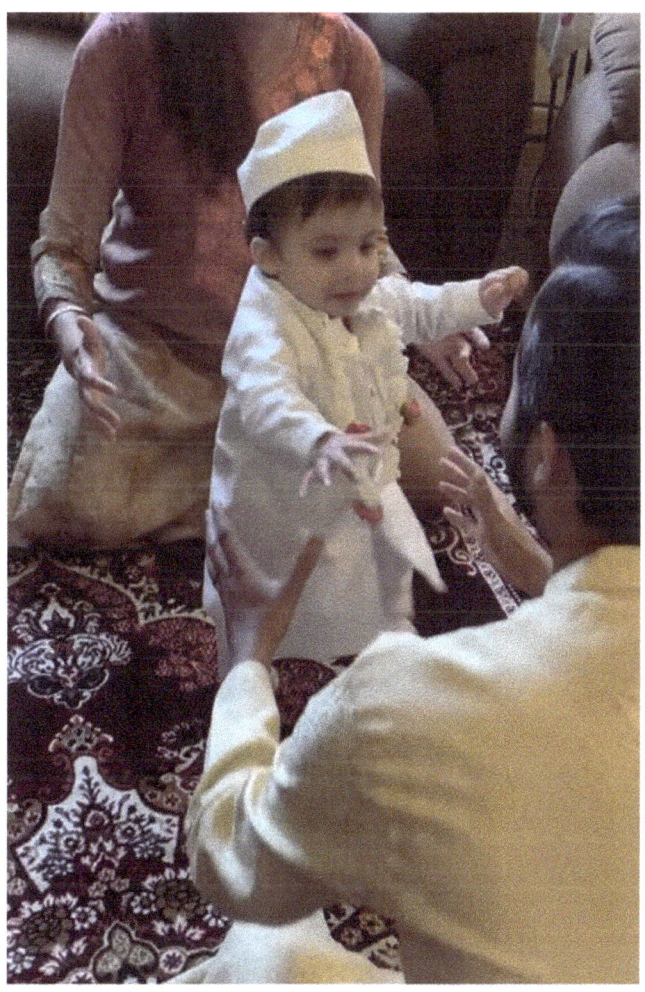

Our son's first steps! Stay close together and don't back up while your baby is in the process of walking. You can slowly increase the distance once your baby has made it to one side. This helps them anticipate the distance and motor plan.

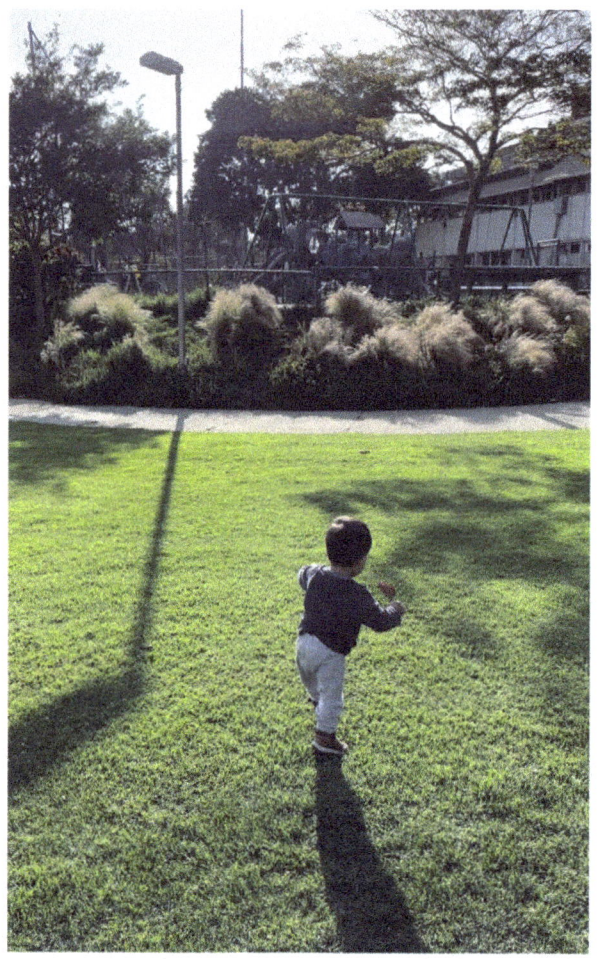

Once your baby is walking, progress their distance and balance by walking on uneven surfaces. Grass is great to challenge balance and for a safer place to fall. Remember, babies who are newly walking fall often. So please make sure the area they are practicing is safe.

Chapter 8

Toys

I wanted to wrap up this book by discussing toys. As mentioned previously, cognition drives motor learning. This means a good toy can motivate your child to start moving and exploring. There are so many toys to consider, so I will discuss qualities to look for in toys for different ages. You may find, as we did, that everyday objects hold more interest than any toy you could buy.

In the first three months, your baby's vision is still limited. Early on, black and white high contrast images will catch their attention. Your baby will develop color vision, first mostly reds and greens. Bright lights and large shapes, especially those that might resemble faces, are more easily seen. Luckily, you can find a lot of board and crinkle books targeted to newborns that have black, white, and red images to catch their attention. Rattles can also be found in these colors and there are plenty of bright light up toys available. Remember that your baby can become over stimulated, so watch their cues when selecting a toy that has bright lights or loud sounds.

As your baby approaches 6 months, they may become more interested in "cause and effect" toys. These are toys that do something in response to some action your baby takes. This often consists of button pushing but could also include things like motion sensors or toys that react to sound. Sensory toys such as crinkle books, water mats, and textured balls will likely hold your baby's interest. Again, light up toys will easily grab their attention. Turning pages of books and banging cups together are simple activities that facilitate fine motor development. Lastly, bubbles and mirrors are easy attention grabbers without providing too much stimulation.

At 9 months, your baby may be on the move crawling. This opens up their world and their access to toys. Toys that allow them to practice this new or emerging skill will pique their interest. You can facilitate crawling over obstacles, like uneven mats or pillows, or crawling through tunnels. Your baby will still be interested in sensory toys, books, cups, and bubbles; and may now expand to musical instruments, like egg shakers and baby pianos, and containers, like food storage containers or tissue boxes. You may find, as we did, that although there are many fancy toys you can purchase to meet these needs, your baby might just prefer the everyday household objects.

By 12 months, your baby is continually expanding their gross and fine motor skills. They may now be interested in pretend play, such as "drinking" out of a play cup. They may start stacking cups and rings, though your baby might be as inclined to knock stacks down. Lastly, your baby is probably captivated by things that open and close, like your cupboards and doors, or if you're lucky, books and play kitchens.

We received so many generous and thoughtful gifts and toys at our baby shower and beyond. Our son loved many of them, but what got the most use were water bottles, food storage containers, mint boxes, cardboard boxes, couch cushions, pillows, leaves, and our mini broom.

Outside of these household items he did play with the stacking cups for a while and loved his books. The toys all had great purpose, but for us, they didn't hold our son's attention for long.

Every child is different and will have different interests, so be ready to hear about the "best toys" that your child has no interest in and try your best to be flexible! If you'd like more recommendations, visit peakplaying.org.

Conclusion

In summary, I hope you use these techniques in your daily play time. Focus on having fun and enjoying the wonder of watching your child grow. Every child is different and will achieve their motor skills in different ways and on different timelines. Having fun with motor play will help your baby continue to explore and enjoy physical activity. If you have concerns, speak with your child's pediatrician, and seek out a pediatric physical therapist consultation.

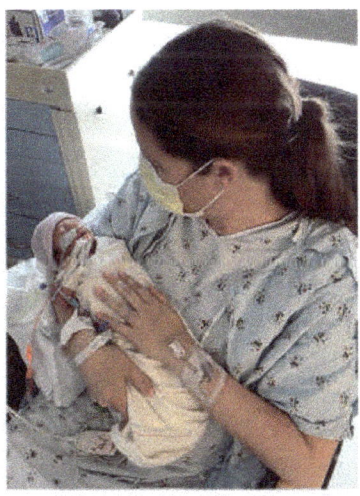

Where he began,
a year before he took his
first steps.

www.ingramcontent.com/pod-product-compliance
Lightning Source LLC
Chambersburg PA
CBHW051546120626
46551CB00013B/1389